Bedside Stories

Michael Foxton is a
doctor working in the NHS.

Bedside Stories

CONFESSIONS OF A JUNIOR DOCTOR

MICHAEL FOXTON

theguardian

Atlantic Books
London

First published in Great Britain in 2003 by Atlantic Books on behalf of Guardian Newspapers Ltd. Atlantic Books is an imprint of Grove Atlantic Ltd.

This rejacketed paperback edition published in 2007 by Atlantic Books on behalf of Guardian Newspapers Ltd.

9 8 7 6 5 4 3

A CIP catalogue record for this book is available from the British Library.

ISBN: 978 1 84354 032 8

Printed and bound in Great Britain by
CPI Antony Rowe, Chippenham, Wiltshire

Atlantic Books
An imprint of Grove Atlantic Ltd
Ormond House
26-27 Boswell Street
London
WC1N 3JZ

This book is dedicated to the glorious socialist republic of the NHS and Alan Milburn, Health Secretary: who angrily denounced doctors as greedy when they rejected his new contract, forcing us into even longer hours, and then resigned to spend more time with his family.

Acknowledgements

Emily Wilson was my editor at The *Guardian*. She is a truly beautiful woman and I loved her dearly. Although, in retrospect, I'm certain she could have paid me much more.

Contents

Introduction

August is a famously good time to stay healthy. The first day I ever worked as a doctor I was on call: walking happily down the corridor, fingering my new bleep, in my white coat, with my stethoscope dangling manfully around my neck. I was feeling strangely competent, when the cardiac arrest bleep went off. These days, of course, I could do an arrest in my sleep – and god knows I've tried often enough – but this time I was on my own and as I looked up I realized I was right outside the ward where all hell was breaking loose. I peered in through the window. No doctors were in sight. On my left there was a toilet and, to my eternal shame, I slipped inside and pretended to have a wee for two minutes. I then dashed on to the ward, bright-eyed and bushy-tailed, after making sure the rest of the team had arrived.

Is that really so bad? It's all about knowing your limitations. Cardiac arrests are strange things. On telly they are the definitive junior doctor moment: everyone sprints heroically to the bedside and bounces up and down on some sweet little old lady's chest as her family look on anxiously, until the angels smile upon her and the little old lady springs miraculously back to life. I hate to be the one to break it to you, but it's just not like that.

Cardiac arrests are ugly and chaotic and they make a mess of a corpse, which is a shame, since the patients never survive anyway and death shouldn't be like that. Later on, during my first night, the registrar introduced me to the concept of the Hollywood call. Families who have watched too many hospital TV dramas occasionally refuse to let the team do the decent thing and put their ageing matriarch 'not for resus'. In preference to arguing the toss and causing distress – and I'll let you be the judge of whether or not it's the right thing to do – it has been known for doctors to opt instead for a Hollywood call. When the patient crashes, the entire cardiac arrest team sprint to the ward, gasping and shouting, bounce up and down on her chest enthusiastically (although delicately enough not to break her ribs) and bark out instructions to each other, giving the stage performance of their lives, before sadly pronouncing to the audience that they did all they could. Do you really need to know this? Probably not. Forget I ever spoke. Stop reading now.

In many ways it was episodes like this that kept me sane. Come on, I think I only ever saw one Hollywood call for real, and they're probably not so awful if you think about it. After all, this sort of thing keeps junior doctors from evacuating the profession in droves. But it's strange how age changes things, because now that I'm quite a good doctor, now that I love my job, and now that I no longer feel persecuted and overworked, reading back through these articles I wonder whether anyone really needs to know what goes on inside the head of a fragmenting junior doctor.

Let me explain: I was working a one in five. This means you work a normal five-day week, but one night in five you work all day, then all night, and then all of the next day. No sleep, hardly eating, constantly walking. It still happens. At the weekend, you start at nine on Saturday and finish on Monday evening. Now, weirdly, this turns out to be perfectly possible, and I suggest you try it if you don't believe me. Your ability to think logically, as far as I can tell, doesn't really tail off, even when your social skills and patience have long since disappeared. But by God, you feel *miserable*. And then you have to deal with the patients.

I have never seen a group of people behave so badly. I know that plenty must have been very nice and polite, although whenever anyone said 'thank you', I almost fell off my legs it was so rare. It's the nasty ones that stick in your memory, I suppose. I know you have to wait for a long time in A&E, and maybe in some hospitals where they can't get permanent nurses it's all very chaotic, and I know you're all ill, but some of what I saw was inexcusable. And it seems to be fashionable to bash doctors everywhere. The newspapers are full of it for a start.

When I was a surgical house officer, I would potter around the ward, explaining the operations to the patients, getting the consent forms signed. They've changed the rules on consenting now, but the principle is the same. People would demand angrily to see the consultant. I would explain that the consultant was in theatre, operating, and that it was my job to explain the operation and his to do it. But they were obsessed with the idea that he was chuckling his way around the golf course or racing through country lanes in his sports car. Some of them even said so. And all this about a man who had devoted his entire life to the NHS, drove a clapped-out banger and regularly stayed until nine at night in the operating theatre, for a quarter of the money he would have got on the continent.

This unthinking rudeness is the thing that's changed the most, and this is the thing that I think older doctors find hardest to understand about junior doctors' working conditions. Nurses have always been a bit mean to junior doctors because they like to get revenge. Fine. But I've talked to older doctors, and they say this: ten years ago, when you told someone you were a doctor at a party, they'd ask if it was really true about the long hours. Now when people find out you're a doctor, they launch into a long and bitter anecdote about how their granny presented passing blood to her GP, and he misdiagnosed her, and she'd still be alive today, if it wasn't for those doctors.

Remember: the NHS is an amazing thing. Only in Britain will you find internationally renowned centres of excellence in the most crack-ridden, poor, radically diverse part of the city.

Although it's all changing now. When you walk into the hospital where I work, you will see a magnificent array of framed portraits, depicting eminent men and women in heroic poses. Who are these noble public servants? This afternoon, for the first time, I wandered over and had a look. Were they eminent surgeons and physicians, nurses, physiotherapists, captured for eternity? No. They were, in fact, the Managers of the Hospital. The people who make me work 70 hours a week, but who themselves go home at five. What heroes. How are you going to survive in a place like this? Find out.

Medical House Officer

The First Six Months

Don't trust me, I'm a new doctor.

This is a very good week to stay well. By the time you read this, as long as it's after 8.30 a.m., I will be a doctor. By which I mean, of course, that I will have started working as one. Since passing my Finals three weeks ago, I have already been a doctor for the purposes of: upgrading my aeroplane seat (unsuccessfully); feeling rather big and clever on my own in a darkened room (incessantly); and impressing my girlfriend (in my dreams).

So now I am left with this hideous mixture of excitement and horror as I slide uncontrollably towards Tuesday morning and come to terms with the fact that I am really going to be a doctor and not a pop star, as previously planned. This is the week that every new doctor in the country starts work in his or her first hospital job. It is a very good week to stay well.

To be honest – and God it pains me – I have never felt so wholly unprepared for anything in my life. Sometimes I worry I only went to medical school to be a nosy parasite. It's a five-year conveyor belt of human experience. I have delivered babies to single mothers with no family support, talked about impotence with builders twice my size and age, and sat chatting to old ladies as they slipped gradually away without a single visit from their relatives; I flatter myself that I've got on pretty well with most of them. What bothers me, though, is those piles of text-books, those endless exams I seemed somehow to have scraped through. I wonder how I can possibly be any more of a doctor than when I left school.

My worry is this: I may well not have been the most diligent medical student ever to don a stethoscope. I assumed it was a clerical error when they read my name out on the pass list. I have, after all, never really 'done' the kidney – and most people have got at least one of those. Surely, please, I must be just the same as any other baby doctor?

If I am not now, I soon will be. My job, like most house officer jobs, is 'compulsorily residential'. I have to live on site, in grim seventies hospital accommodation, surrounded by nothing but other doctors, and far away from the string of friendly shared houses which have been home for the past five years. I only have to stay at work throughout the night a trifling 'one in four' (as we doctors say): it's hard not to see the move as some kind of mind-control strategy. They're trying to cut me off from the normalizing influence of the outside world.

Perhaps I'm just being paranoid. After all, I haven't seen my room, because I can't move in to my warm bed until the evening of my first day on the job, a couple of hours after my unimaginably competent predecessor has moved on. There is, for obvious practical reasons, no rest for the saintly.

But I mustn't grumble; there exists, as far as I can tell, a conspiracy of butchness among doctors, a determination to downplay the heroics. Maybe it all starts to seem pedestrian pretty quickly. And a house officer, too, is plankton, the lowest of the low. Emergencies and stints in casualty excepted, I will be for the most part a highly trained form-filling machine, and even if I do work a 'one in four', that does include four hours of what the contract rather sweetly calls 'semi-protected sleep'.

My desire to conform, to melt into the background and look the part, has never been greater, and so I have been passing my last few days of freedom (seventy hours a week – don't think about it) working on buying myself a proper grown-up doctor's outfit. Something respectable: dashing, but not too showy, maybe a hint of fifties chic – I'm thinking Dirk Bogarde in *Doctor in the House* – to appeal to our older clientele. But all I can find in the department stores are big fat carrot trousers that balloon at the waist and taper at the ankle. I've been a student for five years. These trousers are so hideously far removed from anything I have ever looked for in a pair of pants that I can barely bring myself to force them on to my overdraft.

But in the end, my greatest fear is being left alone. I know they are supposed to handle me with kid gloves. I know that for the first week they are expecting me to be useless. But what about when, as they like to say in medical school Finals, 'your senior cover is busy at an emergency, and you are called to see a man on the ward with chest pains'?

Into the Fray

First I was afraid: I was petrified. My first day at work. You're expecting rivers of blood, piles of corpses. What can I say? I'm touched, but you overestimate the importance of the house officer: the dogsbody in the hospital, a paperwork machine, the enforcer of consultants' whims. My patchy medical knowledge has, in these first two weeks as a doctor, proved mercifully irrelevant.

On my first morning my new consultant (who was so friendly and helpful it was hard not to feel nervous) introduced me and the new senior house officer (SHO) to the registrar – who ignored us all and made for the telephone to discuss a patient in casualty. Twenty seconds later the registrar looked up expectantly; we all fell into line and followed her out onto the ward. I pushed the notes trolley.

During the ward round, the patients were summarized in a sentence, which I scribbled efficiently into my nice new notebook. I ordered every blood test as it was mentioned from a stack of blood forms that I had carefully put in the pocket of my new clipboard, and every other job went into the To Do list on the back. This all gave me an immense sense of achievement and importance.

The consultant and registrar disappeared after the ward round (they always do – no one knows where they go), and the SHO and I worked at our little lists as morning turned into lunchtime.

By the evening, we had almost managed to clear the whole list, but everything seemed to take twice as long as it ought to, nobody wanted to help, and everything needed doing three times over.

No one in the hospital bleeped me back when they said they would, my signature became a scrawl, and my handwriting was going the same way. By 8 p.m. I felt like nothing had quite been finished, but all the other doctors had gone. Feeling inexplicably guilty, I walked the ten yards home, had a microwave meal, and slept like a dead geriatric in my concrete bunker of a bedroom.

On my second day the registrar was unsurprised that half her instructions had gone unenacted, but was appalled to see that no one had written in the patients' notes from yesterday's ward round (her words of wisdom, our management plan). I am the house officer, whose job is defined as everything that is not done by anyone more senior. I apologized and unwisely suggested I could write up yesterday's business today. This, they all pointed out, is vaguely illegal, and the SHO, looking deeply unimpressed, began to write in the notes herself.

The day's jobs trundled by, the previous day's omissions were exposed, and certain recurrent themes began to emerge: the trip down to X-ray (you can send the request form by internal post if you're in the mood, but they just ignore it) and being called by nurses to do bloods on the difficult patients. Everyone, especially the nurses, made it quite clear that I was walking on the eggshells laid down by previous generations of arsey junior doctors. Sucking up to nurses; filling in forms; ordering X-rays: it was mindless bliss. Because I knew what nightmare awaited me that evening.

Ward cover is where they give you six wards with 120 beds, then everyone else goes home for the evening and it becomes your problem. Perhaps that's a little histrionic. Obviously in medicine your ability to obtain senior assistance is limited only by your sense of shame and since I know no shame I am happy to ask for help at every turn. I knew that there was an SHO covering six other wards out there, somewhere on the end of a telephone, but when you answer a bleep on ward cover it is still you, on your own, in a silent hospital with an ill patient, talking to a nurse you've never met.

I am immediately forced to decide on a doctor's manner. Do I adopt a confident yet humble air that will inspire good faith and cooperation – and hide in the toilet to read my pocket textbook of medicine? Or do I risk being busted by pulling it out at the nursing station? I am delighted to find that I seem to know enough medicine to get by on the minor calls: I can tell when Ibuprofen is a good or a bad idea, and I can distinguish the scary causes of nausea from the trivial ones like hospital food, but I still can't quite bring myself to sign my own name on a drug chart without calling my SHO. Even for paracetamol.

My heart only sinks when I am called to review a delirious patient in liver failure. I read the notes and find that she's been in the same appallingly ill state for the past week. It might not be a relief to the patient, but it's a bloody big one for me. I decide to take some bloods to see if she's getting any worse. It's 3 a.m. I dig for a vein and, just as I manage to get one, she starts thrashing her limbs around like a whirling dervish. I try not to freak and hold down her arm, easing out the needle, trying to remember the golden rule for an impending blood squirt: remove the tourniquet, cover your eyes, and close your mouth.

Miffy's First Fuck-up

Today I made the vilest error of my short-lived medical career. It's every newly qualified doctor's nightmare to hear the crash bleep go off and to realize that the call is for a patient on the ward next door – that you will almost certainly be first on the scene; master of ceremonies, however briefly, at the undignified prelude to an inevitable death.

Here's a secret: it also happened on my first day. I was just standing innocently outside 7B waiting for the lift and the crash bleep went off. I looked through the window in the door and there were no doctors in sight. There was no way I was wading in there on my own: I turned around and saw the loo. Of course, I hid.

If you tell anyone, I will find you and kill you. I know how.

But this afternoon, a Sunday, as I sat next to a patient (it was ward cover and I had never seen her before) pondering where best to try and fit a cannula, I heard an almost inaudible sigh. Her posture changed almost imperceptibly and I realized she was dying. No, she was dead.

This is not supposed to be an earth-shattering moment for a medic. At first it seems surprising to patients and medical students alike that anyone could manage to die when they're lying there surrounded by so much technology: a machine to make you breathe; a machine to clean your blood; a cupboard of drugs to sweep away the clots. It had been a long and not entirely incompetent weekend on-call and I had convinced myself I was managing well on my own. So I did my ABC, the mantra of basic life support. Her airway was clear, but there was no breathing and no carotid pulse. And she looked pretty dead to me.

I shifted self-consciously into a managerial role and announced, in what turned out to be my meekest ever English tones: 'Cardiac arrest. Crash team please.' Nurses materialized from nowhere.

'Shall I send out a crash call?' asked a nursing student by the desk.

Well yes, I thought, of course I want a fucking crash call! There is a dead old lady lying here with my tourniquet round her arm. I nodded, business-like and calm, and began my chest compressions while someone fetched a bag and mask and someone else wheeled in the resuscitation trolley.

I heard the call going out on my own bleep. Within ninety seconds doctors began to trickle in. The defibrillator had been watching me from the crash trolley and I had just started wondering if I could really trust myself to use it. But here were the team. They were sweaty but experienced, they were the cavalry, and immediately they asked for the notes and the story. I had been with the patient for ten minutes, long enough to know she needed an IV line, long enough to know from the notes what had happened to her over the past six weeks. I laid out the story and the notes sat on her bedside chair.

Did I mention the relatives? I had forgotten they were there, although it was hard for them not to notice us. This was the moment their beloved mother passed away before their eyes. I, on the other hand, had a patient and a list of things to do. The curtains were pulled and the chest inflations from the bag and mask didn't seem to be doing much. The SHO hurriedly manœuvred a plastic tube down her throat.

There was no pulse and there was 'no reversible cause'. The defibrillator electrodes were on and the monitor showed ventricular fibrillation. *VF is the commonest pulseless electrical activity*, I thought inanely, from the facts burned into my brain, *and the one that is most frequently shockable*. I could even give you the page reference for that one. A line was placed in both arms and the anaesthetist began struggling to get one into her neck. I allowed myself to be sidelined.

'OK, I'm ready to shock. All clear.'

It is the responsibility of the person who administers the shock to ensure everyone is clear, the voice of ancient revision recited in my ear. The patient was obviously very dead . . . 200 volts and she arched into the air. Check: no pulse, no change, VF . . . 200 volts, she jolted: no pulse, no change, except this time a wheeze as the air was forced out of her chest . . . 360 volts.

Perhaps I'm not explaining myself properly. What I was watching was horrific: wires in her neck, tubes in her throat, spasms of electrocution. It may even have been painful. It certainly sounded like it from the cracking ribs as we bounced up and down on her chest between shocks. It was undignified and traumatic and the routine cycled around for what felt like an hour.

Registrars come to arrests to tell you when to stop. Ours came and took one look at the notes, one little look at the NOT FOR RESUSCITATION pink form – ticked, signed and dated six weeks before, reviewed every week, a form marked NOT FOR RESUSCITATION: ON GROUNDS OF FUTILITY, ON GROUNDS OF QUALITY OF LIFE.

Ticked – but unnoticed by me. Discussed with nurses, discussed with medical staff, discussed with patient, discussed with relatives, every last one was ticked. So there I stood, thinking: Am I guilty of assault or abuse of a corpse? Was it a crime against this woman or her family? Was it my fault?

Obviously.

I knew nothing about this woman. I just marched in at the end with the fireworks at the most acutely personal moment of her long life. *If there is any doubt about resuscitation status, you must always put out a crash call*. I don't care. This is the worst thing I have ever done.

Bugs with Wings

I think I've gone native. Three weeks ago I'd have ducked for cover if a patient sneezed on me: today I almost forgot to wash my hands after a rectal examination on a constipated diabetic, and my generally jovial manner took a bit of a bashing when the rota coordinator called to tell me about a little error they had made before we arrived, which somehow involves me working next Saturday at less than a week's notice. There was, needless to say, a brief moment of self-righteousness on my part (one day I even went home before 6 p.m.), but I've been struggling to keep this corrosive bitterness at bay. They don't make it easy.

To my astonishment, after six weeks I've started to get a feel for who is ill and who is not, and the first thing to realize is that there are plenty of people in hospital who are an awful lot healthier than you or me. They stay here because there seems to be a vast army of patients, relatives, and social workers who all labour under the delusion that hospital is a safe place to be if you are old and healthy with nowhere to go. It's not.

Once you're here we give you all the horrible infections that the patient two beds away came in with, plenty of which will only be treated with the antibiotics that we will invent in the year 2007: until then you die – after you've had diarrhoea from the antibiotics we do have, which then throws off your mental functioning and, before you know it, you can't make it to the loo on your own any more and you're on the month-long waiting list for a nursing home. I do my bit by washing my hands between patients, but as far as I can tell these bugs have wings. For their sake, get your parents out of hospital as fast as you can.

The other thing they tend not to mention in the textbooks is that nothing works like they say in the textbooks. For example: there are fifty year olds who cycle to work every day and then there are fifty year olds who smoke in front of the telly, and they all get ill in pretty much the same way. And I go through this painfully thorough clerking routine on every patient I see in casualty, but still, for anything other than the barn-door classics like strokes, the patterns of symptom and sign have nothing to do with anything I ever studied in medical school. Presumably I'm doing something wrong. And more than anything, whatever their problem is, you can always kind of see the ones that are going to be fine and the ones that are in for the distance, from the moment you walk into the cubicle.

The strange thing is, despite my crippling lack of confidence (but you should see me exuding the stuff), the more I am left alone the more competent I seem to become. My consultant is away at a conference. My SHO is on nights. I do ward rounds on my own, I make management decisions that even my monster of a research registrar (the nice one is on holiday) manages not to publicly ridicule, and sometimes I do a bit of good. Even the stroppiest nurses have stopped treating my requests for a quick set of patient observations as a class-war issue.

Ah, stroppiness: sometimes it feels like it's everywhere around me, and the worst of it is that I have become a purveyor of the stuff myself, despite my better judgement. It's the inescapability of the work. What were previously isolated little puddles of labour seem to be joining up into vast oceans of drudgery and I never seem to be away from the hospital for more than four hours at a time. I live in a small concrete bunker fifteen yards from my ward, and whenever I go home from a night out I have to walk past the main doors of the casualty department.

With this – together with the all-nighters in casualty every five days and the time-warp effect of spending your every moment on and off the job in a hospital that never sleeps – the days just merge into one another. I used to pride myself on being pretty good at sleep deprivation, but that was when I was a student and I could award myself a day off to recover after a heavy revision session. This is relentless, inescapable exhaustion, and it's all made so much worse by my churlish refusal to ditch my social life.

But whenever I do manage to escape into the real world, I can't get over how young and healthy you all look. I bet most of you can even make it to the toilet on your own. It just makes me want to be one of you again. So be kind to me, please, and remember what I said about the bugs: keep yourself out of hospital, and don't go after a doctor in the queue for the canteen salad bar.

Lost, Alone, Afraid and Despised

I'm beginning to suspect that I just cannot cope. I know I'm supposed to be having an awful time, I know it's part of the job and it's not as bad as it used to be – as every doctor over fifty proudly points out – but this is real, this is me. I'm a real person and eight weeks ago I was a normal person and now I feel lost and alone and afraid and incompetent and out of my depth and universally despised for it by every nurse and patient I talk to.

The house officer on the next ward got a bladder infection last week from under-hydrating herself: what kind of ridiculous job do I have when the best advice your colleagues can offer is to eat whenever you possibly can, because you never know what might happen next, and make sure you watch your urine output? She treated herself with Augmentin – a sledgehammer – and was delighted to find that geriatric patients aren't the only ones to get green mucous diarrhoea from the stuff. The moral is to take drugs seriously. Junkies kindly take note, and stop waking me up at 3 a.m. to ask for pethidine you obviously don't need.

God, it's tough. I get things wrong: I forget to do things. I run through the patients in my head when I'm at the cinema and compulsively phone the ward from my mobile to check I haven't messed up anything and killed anyone. God, I'm so hysterical – none of them are really that ill. No matter how many lists and counter-lists I write in my little file I always mess up something – only little things. Honestly. Teeny things. Like pursuing a scan report that would arrive by itself in two days anyway. But it makes me feel like a blubbery idiot on the verge of tears when my consultant asks me for the results on the ward round and I just don't know them.

Of course I don't know them. I have to look them up. Nobody knows them. Anybody would have to look them up. But how can I begin to expect you to understand how shit I've been feeling about myself when I don't even believe the other house officers when they start whingeing? I grumble and moan and they all tell me it's the same for everyone, but I just can't believe it. They all look so swish.

So have I become moody? Do I snap? No. I have reinvented myself as a slightly hysterical over-friendly ball of energy that bounces from one patient to the next, saying 'Hell-o, sir!' in an irritating, sing-song happy-camper voice and repressing my anxiety and fear by multi-tasking like Shiva on amphetamines with three drug charts, six blood forms and five sets of notes spread across my nine pairs of hands. And I've been fantasizing about fitting my white coat (by God, do I look cool in it) with a few huge auxiliary pockets, and a shoulder-mounted tank of nebulized Ventolin to spray on to the endless stream of asthmatics who pile in through casualty.

At least they've fixed the heating in my crappy hospital room, although the radiator is burning hot and attached to the only wall long enough to have a bed against it (and I still need to close the door to open the wardrobe and pull out another unironed shirt). Fatigue enhances the effects of the cold, but I still need to keep the window open to fumigate the airborne residue left behind by my stinky predecessor. Right now I'm shivering in two jumpers and trying to believe it's not just the caffeine.

The worst of it all was when my research registrar spent three whole days systematically pointing out to me and the consultant how shit I am at my job, before buggering off to some clever conference and leaving me alone on the ward with thirty patients. By my maths (and I've only been a doctor for two months) someone with eight years' experience has precisely fifty-two times as much experience as me. I find this kind of ritual public flogging fantastically unhelpful.

So, in the military hierarchy of medicine I have resorted to the only form of catharsis available to me: I take it out on anyone I can find who is more junior than me. You think I've been bullying nurses? God, you're sick: I mean medical students. But half of them seem to know more medicine than I do. I give up and take them to see a guy who lost his memory when he lost his liver (booze) and has now started confabulating. He doesn't have a clue what's going on around him, but fills in the gaps with some rather imaginative nonsense. He has an answer for everything. ('Sound familiar, Michael?' asked my registrar when he first demonstrated the phenomenon.)

The patient refuses to play ball, however, and seems perfectly oriented and alert. I shrug and lead my troops away from the bed. As we walk away the patient suddenly looks up chirpily and shouts out: 'Oh, and when are we docking, Captain?'

Quite.

The Power of One

I'm beginning to work out what's wrong with all those TV hospital dramas: the characters are never on their own. When they're not flirting over the defibrillator pads, they're debating some burning ethical issue behind the nursing station or tenderly consoling each other over a cup of vending-machine soup.

On the whole, they tend not to depict junior doctors on ward cover at 3 a.m. wondering what the hell they're going to do with a patient who's spiking a temperature that's been ignored all day – on unfamiliar wards staffed by bank nurses who have no interest in even looking at you, let alone showing you where the patient is.

Just to be extra helpful, most hospitals have now abolished that nice big white board behind the nurses' desk that has the patients' names on it, having anticipated several months ago (bizarrely) that it might infringe future human rights legislation on privacy. This costs me – and anyone else who sees patients on unfamiliar wards – an average of one minute's pissing about for every patient seen, which works out at four minutes an hour or one hour in a shift or a fifth of my projected sleeping time on an average night of ward cover. I lie awake at night on-call performing angry calculations on sleep deprivation. Believe me, I could bore for England on the subject.

To be fair though, I rather enjoy pootling around the wards on my own, sorting out people here and there and acting as a unilateral medical force (especially since it's the only time I feel like a doctor rather than a paperwork clerk). Although your average TV scriptwriter would have to work pretty hard to derive any narrative tension from my little wanders, particularly now that I have perfected my air of inscrutable, calm professionalism in the face of nauseous exhaustion.

Perhaps that's why no one takes me seriously when I whinge about being tired: or maybe we've all just used up our whinge credits. Perhaps that's why even the nicer nurses will cheerily say something really unhelpful like 'You chose the hours when you chose the job.'

Empathy, it must be said, is a problem that cuts both ways. So, last night I was called to see a patient who was pretty obviously about to die. Having established this ball-park diagnosis (largely by exclusion: there was no way she was going to live) and anxiously double-checked it with my SHO, I shared the unhappy news with the family. It was, if I say so myself, a moment even our dismal communication skills lecturer would have been proud of. It certainly compared favourably to my previous 'breaking bad news' moment, when I had just been called from bed and was wearing theatre trousers and a borrowed T-shirt that said SHEFFIELD MEDICS AT YOUR CERVIX.

I retreated to the wards, leaving the family to do their business (and a lot of the stuff in the last few hours is business) and five hours later I was bleeped to be told that the patient was dead. Now, of course, my heart skipped: I don't know if I watched too many cop shows when I was a kid, but for some reason I can't shake the idea that a dead body is somehow a legal issue, until proven otherwise. Every corpse should have its own explanation, legitimizing and permitting an unruly death, and in this case that explanation was me.

A real live dead person. On my head. Only a few people had seen this woman alive, except for her adoring family who had noddingly swallowed the improvised platitudes I downloaded for them on my way to a rushed lunch. Suddenly, out of nowhere, for no reason, I panicked: Inspector Columbo was definitely on the way.

Shit, I thought, for one fleeting moment. I've got a fucking corpse on my hands.

Now in times like these, there is always an entry in the *Hands on Guide for House Officers* (holy tome, we are not worthy). The weirdest learning curve of becoming a doctor is when you realize that words in books translate into actions in the real world, which themselves translate into tangible impacts on the mortality of the person lying in bed in front of you; a chain of cause and effect that has only recently begun to seem plausible to me.

I look up DEATH and am pleasantly surprised to find one definitive entry. There's a string of platitudes about not letting it freak you out, which I ignore – until I remember that I've only looked up what to do with dead people because I've got one right in front of me that is properly freaking me out. I stop freaking out. And then it turns out that all there is left to do is the pronouncement of death. Which all looks pretty easy: I put it to the back of the queue and start working through my backlog of bleep calls.

So you're waiting for the punchline? Nothing more than an act of crass thoughtlessness, I'm afraid. After six hours that felt like five minutes, running between crappy half-pneumonias and writing up interminable IV fluids, I'm bleeped again and finally make it up to the ward to find an entire family waiting expectantly for me to place the seal on their mum's death. And for a fleeting, exhausted moment, would you believe, I was even miffed that they'd been impatient?

Sort of Sorted

You catch me at a bit of a bad moment. I mean, if you've been paying any attention to what I've been telling you over the past ten weeks (wow, check out how impatient I've become), you are probably under the impression that my whole life is an unending series of bad moments: death, disease, dishonour, dismay, and all the other junior doctor stuff. But that's not true. I've worked it all out now: it only seems shit when you're not there.

So, on Sunday morning, after two nights of four hours' sleep, after the weekend when winter came early for the relentlessly diseased inhabitants of our catchment area – a weekend which I had accidentally started with a hangover – my skin was blotchy, my eyes were red, my head was throbbing, and I was in seventh heaven.

I had seen dozens of patients, two of them were kicking off simultaneously before my very eyes so one of them was definitely my problem, and I was loving every second. Every nurse was my friend, every vein caught first time, and the symptoms and signs were arranging themselves into neat little frameworks of recognizable pathology.

I might not have been the best doctor in the world, but I was there in the fray, coping with my job, running through protocols and affecting an air of empathic sensitivity while feeling pretty fucking butch, I can tell you.

Whereas right now I am sitting at a kitchen table in the flat of my oldest friend, digesting some home-cooked food, listening to a record, smoking a cigarette, surrounded by home comforts, and I feel dismal. This coming weekend, another on-call (by a cruel accident of our insane rota) hangs over me like a threat. I am watching the clock and calculating exactly how little sleep I can get away with and still function tomorrow.

I'd be OK if the outside world didn't exist.

I guess what you really want to hear about are disasters. I shan't oblige. To a frail mortal like me, all this When Doctors Kill business on the telly is a bit demoralizing. But let me at least furnish you with a paradox: I discover to my astonishment that I am not the most pointless person in the hospital.

On Saturday, casualty was knee-deep. They were crawling up the walls in the waiting room, so our consultant, demonstrating a breathtakingly egalitarian outlook, grabbed the fresh new medical student and announced that he would go and clerk in a couple of the new patients.

There are two things that should immediately strike you as odd about this scenario. First, the fact that there is a medical student in the hospital on a Saturday morning at all is something I find intensely threatening. When I was a student, Saturday (much like Friday and Monday) was a day of rest.

Second, consultants do not clerk patients. God knows what else they do. They write papers on diseases that no one ever gets. They float in once a week and spend two hours being nice to you about all the easy patients you have subjected to your own inimitable brand of mediocre management. They sit in committee meetings (I am told) comparing their immense private-practice pay cheques under the table, chuckling over the Government's new rules for incoming consultants which state that they must do NHS work exclusively for the first seven years of their contract, and roaring with laughter over the extra clientele this will bring them.

My own consultant, uniquely, takes his juniors aside for little chats every now and then. You feel that, if you really wanted to, you could probably tell him that you cry in the toilets on the ward about once a week and he would have some sound advice to offer on the subject. Consultants do not clerk patients in the casualty department.

So anyway, three hours later the consultant emerged from the cubicle and calmly announced that everything was in hand. (In fact he used the word 'sorted', which I guess he must have picked up from the streetwise teenage medical student.) No one dared or thought to question him. The patients continued to clamour at the windows outside.

Three hours later, it turned out that the patient the consultant had seen had had no blood tests done, no drug chart, no chest X-ray, no medication, and no bed booked. And here, finally, I saw that I do have my own humble little place in the world after all, as our proud leader strode confidently off out of casualty: 'This medicine lark, you know, endlessly fascinating. I've forgotten more than I ever knew.'

What I Really Do for a Living

Apparently horses can sleep standing up with their eyes open. Now here's what really aggravates me: all the other people in the hospital who aren't doctors, but who look after the same patients as me, go home at 5 p.m. every day. Occupational therapists, physiotherapists, speech and language therapists, clinical nutrition specialists, ward clerks, X-ray secretaries, social workers, phlebotomists: with a few honourable exceptions, they are very careful to make an extremely sharp exit. They plan their day around it. It wouldn't occur to them to stay, like I do, until 6.30, often beyond eight, until the patients are 'sorted'. It just wouldn't.

Once they leave the building – bang on time – two things happen. First, if the job they should have done is urgent, I stay behind and do it myself. Nice. Alternatively, if the job isn't urgent (like a home visit to assess someone for services), the patient just sits around in hospital for another few days waiting to catch a hospital-acquired infection that will knock them right over and be resistant to all known antibiotics.

Meanwhile there are patients sleeping on trolleys in casualty.

Now there are a lot of reasons why junior doctors are made to feel guilty for complaining about their long hours. The therapists I listed above will tell me that I chose the hours when I chose the job (when I was at school aged seventeen, I suppose) and they all reckon I'm going to be so loaded when I grow up that I deserve to have a shit life now.

Thanks.

Sometimes they'll start laying into me about my future riches if I happen to mention that I'm feeling a bit rough after three hours' sleep (when really I mean 'tearful'). Usually it's just as they're rushing out to catch the 4.55 train home and telling me about the things they've 'not been able to fit in' that day. I'm determined not to start thinking they're all arseholes. I guess they feel undervalued.

Consultants – who, of course, worked even more ridiculous hours in their day – will tell you that doctors need to accumulate clinical experience for their professional training, and that this takes time. Which would all be very well if I spent my days practising clinical medicine, but – as I may have already mentioned about eight million times – in the daytime on the wards (as opposed to when I'm on-call) I am a paperwork clerk, a machine for processing forms, a robot for carrying them from A to B, a St Bernard for seeking out lost X-rays in the radiology department, and a mobster's enforcer for bullying social workers into sorting out my patients.

None of these useful learning opportunities will help me get my membership of the Royal College of Physicians in two years' time. I love being on-call, even all night. I would dearly love to work as a doctor, day in, day out, to absorb myself in the healing arts. If you took out all the parts of my job that should be done by someone else – like a ward secretary maybe – and left me just doing the doctor stuff, on some days I'd be home by lunchtime. Then I could leave work early after being up all night on-call. Or you could give me more patients to learn from. Either would be great.

But there is another, darker reason why we have to work such long hours. Just as the other health professionals in the hospital know that they can ultimately rely on doctors to sort out the patients if they'd rather go home on time, so do the managers of the hospital trust. Why would an organization like a hospital, run by managers, want to employ an extra ward clerk or a phlebotomist to take the bloods, for £5 an hour, when a doctor will stay late and do it for free? There isn't a manager alive who wouldn't take an opportunity like that to screw me over.

Up and down the country this week, small conspiratorial bands of junior doctors were crouched in their squalid underground bunkers filling out their 'banding questionnaires' to work out which pay scale their job will fall into. I don't know anyone who won't fall into the top one (more than fifty-six hours a week), although I know about plenty of hospitals that are trying to bribe and bully their doctors into lying on the form.

So doctors will continue to work their ridiculous hours, albeit for money, but its not the money we're in the game for: that money is going to hit those cold-hearted scumbags who manage hospitals and make us work seventy-hour weeks right where it hurts and make them do something about it.

Because the pay for each band increases exponentially in relation to the lunacy of the workload, doctors will suddenly become more expensive than other staff. And two doctors working seventy-five hours each will cost more than three happy doctors working fifty. Doctors will finally get the deal they deserve, not through anyone's sense of decency and humanity, but only because cash is the only language hospital managers understand.

The Animal in Us

Patients are like wild animals: you can never show fear or they will attack. I'm tempted to believe that we have a habit of over-complicating things, not just to patients but to each other, in order to bolster an illusory sense of control and keep everyone sane. On some level, even to the most educated and interested patient, we routinely lie in our mannerisms and attitudes, because medicine isn't a precise business; and if you took a moment to be honest with yourself, patients would admit that they find it hard to cope with that, especially when your mortality is hitting you in the chest for the first time in your imperilled life, and especially in Accident and Emergency (A&E).

You don't want me standing over you in casualty thinking out loud: 'Buggered if I know, but you can't die too quickly as long as I hit you with some oxygen and keep your circulation moving.' You want nurses and doctors dashing in and out of the cubicle, barking out coded instructions with thinly veiled urgency: you want the machine that goes *ping!*, you want to be seen the moment you walk in the door, and you want it all to happen to the soundtrack of a drum-and-bass remix of the *Casualty* theme tune.

What you get, of course, after waiting for several hours in a crowded waiting room full of screaming toddlers and haemorrhaging tramps, is a junior doctor like me. And once I've ascertained that you're not on the verge of death – while you're sizing me up for the haggard-looking teenager I appear to be (I promise you, I'm twenty-four and I work well under pressure) – I'm trying to figure out what kind of doctor you want me to be, because most of the time it's harder than diagnosing your (rather pedestrian) angina attacks.

The stakes are high. I've had patients – who were either demented or plain belligerent – just clam up on me: I swear, I was so friendly and relaxed that they just stopped taking me seriously and waited for a real doctor to arrive. I may feel the same way myself sometimes but, believe me, those real doctors can take a very long time to answer their bleeps. I know I can't expect it to be any other way. I can't expect you to tick the box marked AUTHORITARIAN MEDICAL PRACTITIONER PLEASE any more than I expect you to fall out of the ambulance with SUBDURAL HAEMATOMA – SCAN MY HEAD PLEASE written on your T-shirt.

But what I don't like is when it gets complicated and you uppity, over-educated *Guardian* readers get all bitchy because I'm not telling you exactly what diagnostic options are passing through my head; then you demand an extensive treatise on exactly why your ninety-seven-year-old mother fell off the commode this morning, when the best I can come up with is that her house is a mess, the telephone cable is spangled across the room at ankle height, she can't see without her specs, and her children should frankly have done the honourable thing and either put her in a home or let her move in with them in their flash central London *pied-à-terre*.

Am I ranting? I apologize. Just try to remember that if you're going to die on the doorstep, we'll save you if anyone can – and if you're not, then we're doing just fine, *Holby City* histrionics or not. This is a teaching hospital for God's sake: we spew out doctors faster than you spew up blood. This is as good as it gets.

On a more important note, I'd like to share with you my research findings on the transmissibility and infective nature of body odour. My interest was first aroused when the groins on one particular geriatrics ward started smelling the same as that of Mr P., a relatively new arrival to our surreal little salon, but two wards away. He had been festering in an acute medical bed at risk of hospital-acquired infections, while social services quietly ignored him, for a trifling three weeks.

Body odours, as far as I can tell, are the result of a peculiar interplay between the nutrients secreted in your body's natural juices and the microbes that feed on them. Just as different species of bacteria and fungi have furnished the French with a wide variety of cheeses from the same kind of milk, so a different selection of invisible helpers seem to be at work in the armpits, gussets, and insoles of us all. This is an area in which I have recently become something of a connoisseur.

At first the aroma of condensed egg white and vinegar was confined to the other gentlemen sharing Mr P.'s bay, whose sores had been tended by the same team of nurses. Within a week it had spread throughout the male end of the ward and recently we have been detecting it on the surgical wards three floors below. And now, this morning, as I sit in my towel waiting for the doctor with whom I share a bathroom to finish his interminable shower, I cannot ignore the heady, familiar aroma that drifts up from my own groin and fills my nostrils. This is not a chain of events on which I want to dwell.

Death Wishes

Medicine has taken over my entire field of vision. I can't look at my girlfriend's forearms without thinking how easy and satisfying it would be to gently slip a cannula into her prominent, lovely veins. When we kiss, I'm feeling up her spine and assessing the best place to insert a lumbar puncture needle. I've managed to cut down on calling the ward from my mobile after work, but I can't stop making diagnoses on the bus.

You will be relieved to hear that we have all been washing our hands with unswerving diligence, which is more than I can say for some of our patients – one of whom I interrupted this morning urinating in his NHS water jug because his bottle was full. People on the cusp of dependence, I suspect, don't like asking for help, and I can see a lot of myself in some of the things they do, which I suppose is why I like them. I guess that's also why I felt particularly awkward on his behalf when the consultant came back from answering a call and poured him out a glass of water, explaining that he had to keep drinking if we were ever going to take down his drip. Needless to say we (me and the patient) kept our mouths shut.

Death and disease continue unabated, but self-inflicted suffering seems to be all the rage among the patients coming my way in casualty this month. Teenage suicide attempts are always a treat, because (like deep-vein thromboses) they're quick to manage and a good way to keep your numbers up in A&E. There's nothing like a reputation for ploughing through patients and clearing the waiting list in the run-up to the Christmas rush.

Junkies, on the other hand, are a different story. First of all, let me put my cards on the table. As a *Guardian*-reading liberal wet I tend to believe that heroin addicts are victims of society and that their victimization is counter-productive, the source of most of their problems, and emblematic of us victimizing the morally weak in society in general.

Which is all very well until they steal my video recorder or pitch up in casualty at 1 a.m. covered in vomit. Opiate overdoses, in the textbook, are very easy to manage: you hit them with an antidote called naloxone and, frankly, it would be easier if they just handed out the stuff at needle exchanges and saved us all the bother.

Now I don't know if you've ever looked at the arms of your average junkie, but by the time they get in deep enough to overdose, they've usually knocked off every vein in their body. The company they keep tends to be friendly to the point of total disinhibition, and their companions are always eager to get involved in the workings of the casualty department. I'm always tempted to ask for their help getting into a vein, because I imagine that they're far better at it than me.

The other thing that textbooks tend not to mention about giving naloxone is that the moment it kicks in the patient kicks out and sits up bolt upright, bright-eyed and bushy-tailed, demanding to know what the fuck you think you are doing, wasting £10 worth of prime smack he worked really very hard for, and then shouts his head off for half an hour. Then, just when you are about to get away, the antidote wears off, they slip back into respiratory arrest and start trying to choke on their own vomit again. This is no fun at all.

But the worst thing is that people just keep on trying to die on me, against the best efforts of everyone around them. So on Thursday night I had yet another family trying to blackmail me into shoving tubes in to feed their dying matriarch who, despite speaking not a word of English, was very clearly both well-oriented and determined to pass away peacefully (and thank God it was a weeknight, so I could safely leave the decision for her own team to make the next morning).

And this morning a man I had looked after for three weeks, whom I had caught laughing at the newspapers every morning ('It's all just a load of nonsense; I'm so glad I'm leaving it all behind'), who sat me down the first time we met in A&E and somehow made me share all my aspirations with him before telling me that I had it all wrong, that the most important thing in life was the person you chose to spend it with, and that when his wife of fifty-three years had passed away he knew he was going to follow her soon . . . this morning he finally willed himself to death.

A Failure to Care

Prepare yourself for an orgy of unbridled self-pity and loathing. I'm not proud of the person I've become: because I'm everything you predicted I would be.

Callous? Maybe I'm just overfamiliar with misery, panic and pain. People don't die every day (although the guy in the mortuary who bleeps with terrible monotony to get me to sign death certificates thinks he's being pretty funny when he calls me Dr Shiplake), but if they're not ill and in intractable pain, then they've been abandoned by their families or they're desperate to be discharged, and there's never much I can do apart from smile, which I am doing less and less.

I am gradually, regrettably, ceasing to care. I bet the man who runs the roller-coaster at Alton Towers doesn't get scared when he goes on it for the hundredth time. But I feel like I should be involved in my patients' pain – and the relatives do too: if I'm not concerned, if I'm not astonished and aghast at the sheer scale of their appalling ill-health to the point of devoting myself to twenty-four-hour bedside supervision, then they make no effort to hide their disappointment.

Part of the problem is, of course, that I'm just so busy.

'What was the result of that test my father had yesterday, doctor?' people ask, quite reasonably. And the responses that spring into my head, in order of increasing shamefulness, are: 'What test?', 'How the fuck should I know?' and 'What's it got to do with you?' And when I'm not cursing families for pestering me, I'm cursing them for dumping their grannies on the doorstep.

Which brings me on to Christmas and my own special appeal. Don't dump your granny on me this Christmas. In fact, please could you try especially hard not to dump them on either Christmas Eve or 27 December, the days when I'm working in

A&E. The 27th, it might amuse you to know, has been statistically demonstrated as the worst day in the year for granny-dumping, and will be particularly horrific this year, after a long weekend with no GP surgeries.

And all that anyone ever wants to talk about is medicine: my friends, my mum, even my patients. I wandered into a patient's room for a quick chat the other night, during a quiet moment on ward cover and all I was seeking was a bit of solace and a quiet moment. I even offered him some lemon cordial: he's a nice guy, we get on well, and he knows a lot about old movies. But as soon as I get in there, all he can talk about is his endless afflictions.

The thing I'm not telling you is that I just want to get out. I don't have the nerve, the commitment, the staying power, the moral reserve, the social skills, the competitiveness, the caring nature, the backbone – I just don't have any of that stuff you need to be a doctor. I feel awful at least ten times a day. I cry at least once a week (and I'm a boy). I tell my senior house officer and all she can do is smile and say 'You'll feel like that more than you can ever possibly imagine, for years and years.'

What do they think they're all playing at? They're all either heavy drinkers or compulsively unfaithful or addicted to the gym – or in one case masturbation (a drunken confession). Doctors talk about the crap lifestyle of hospital medics as if a pleasant lifestyle were slightly camp or incidental or disposable. But junior doctors have no lifestyle outside of being doctors, and most of our patients are geriatric nightmares with nothing more than social problems, getting worse and worse the longer they spend in hospital.

So think of me and my abysmal self-pity when you're having fun this year around the Christmas tree, and remember our special appeal [*Terry Wogan Children-in-Need voice, stirring music, soft-focus footage of old ladies gambolling gaily in the garden*]: 'Keep them at home this Christmas.'

White Coat, Black Heart

I often think about how we keep families out of the resuscitation room in A&E. How the sight of their dying father with a triple-bore central line sticking out of his blood-soaked neck, his groin betraying the scars of my traumatic practice runs at inserting a femoral arterial line, his chest, covered in electrode pads, being used as a coffee table for bits of equipment, and his trousers lying in half on the trolley beneath him . . . how it all might be too disturbing for the relatives.

To be honest, the sound of them in tears outside the door, demanding to be let in, is often the only thing that can bring home what exactly is unfolding before me, and that alone feels like a good enough reason not to let them in, because you don't want to think about that kind of thing when the registrar is barking out instructions and you're trying to get arterial blood gases off quickly enough to impress the anaesthetist so that he'll talk you through the next patient's femoral arterial line (get to do a few yourself, it looks great on the CV).

Gradually, by subterfuge, these episodes are changing me, or at least cleaving off my work persona from the boy next door I imagine I must still be. The process of depersonalization that starts in casualty is just as real on the wards. You cannot rely on innate charm with patients at 3 a.m., and you cannot afford to take it personally when that notoriously unhelpful nurse on 7E starts bouncing up and down and giving you grief about somebody else's blood form. You have to learn to not give a shit.

Sometimes I am astonished to catch myself on autopilot, asking nothing but pertinent questions (I kid you not), smiling away, almost completely unaware of the fact that I am talking to a person and not a box with QUERY UNSTABLE ANGINA written on its forehead, who may or may not need IV isoket and heparin, depending on how highly it scores on the tick list in my head. The rare occasions when I offend or cause distress are the times when I am foolish enough to chance my luck at just being myself instead of a robot.

But the strangest thing is that this hugely effective depersonalization of the patients, this reinvention of myself as a walking bedside manner, is exactly what I have started to do to myself as the only way to stave off the powerful inner drive towards self-pity and resentment of the NHS and how it has ruined my life.

It is a resentment that has cut even deeper over the festive period, when everyone else is at home watching *It's a Wonderful Life* on the sofa with their mum and dad, and the only way to cope is to make yourself love the job by buying into the delusory self-sacrificing herd mentality of junior doctors where nothing outside the hospital matters any more, where you do not expect to have a life, where friends are a thing of the past, where disasters are a challenge and where you have to love your work because to expect anything more from life is to court disappointment.

So this is what I have learned this year, more than how to manage myocardial infarction: how to stop the patients from punishing me, how to cope with evil politics on the ward, and how to stop taking it as a personal affront or judgement on my character when a patient falls ill.

If I grit my teeth hard enough, the festive period (which was anything but) was a delight. A&E was full to boiling the day after Boxing Day, and the casualty sister was sending patients up to the admissions ward (about a million miles away, since you ask) before they had even been seen. Each and every one of them was a social and medical disaster zone, neglected by all and sundry for the whole of the preceding week, and there was nothing we could do for most of them but admit them to our Geriatric Hotel. These people are sent to punish us. Let them come. Our admissions list, previously an index of pain, went on to a fifth page, and we loved it.

I have become a medic. I have put on my blinkers, drawn up my galoshes, and waded into the bloodbath before me. The

patients over the four-day-long Christmas holiday were under-
hydrated and grossly mismanaged, dry as a crisp: it wasn't my
fault, but, better than that, it was a great opportunity to practise
my central line technique.

Just a Little Prick

'What's the polar opposite of being shafted by the NHS?'

That's how my SHO announced that she was ditching me
for the world of investment banking. The move, like everything
else she has ever done, was exercised with almost military pre-
cision. I know that baby doctors tend to mythologize the
superhuman powers of their immediate superiors. We are, after
all, dependent on them for matters of life and death and they
can pull some pretty amazing stuff out of the bag sometimes.
This was no exception: a study week, scrounged for membership exams, she spent on work experience with Mammon
himself; a twenty-book reading list of unrelenting tedium
before the interview; swotting the financial pages every day for
a year on the way to work. I don't know where she gets the
energy. Oh, yes I do.

'In my new company,' she said, 'when you work late, they get
you a taxi home.' We were walking back over to the concrete
bunker where they keep the junior doctors at night. It was 2 a.m.
'If you're going to miss dinner, they arrange for food to be delivered from the restaurant downstairs.' She waved at the vending
machine full of instant meals (dry ones that don't even need
refrigerating) that lives at the bottom of our staircase, as we wandered in to the mess. 'And they have a gym in the basement and
a swimming pool full of money.'

We started fantasizing about having our own house-officer
butlers.

'A call from 7E, sir, on the other side of the hospital. Shall I
fetch your carriage around?'

'Yes, Jeeves, and this coffee's a bit shit. Send down to the kitchen will you old boy?'

But my heart was heavy with loss.

My first SHO is leaving me, I thought, as we sat in the squalor of the mess. But I will never forget the way she helped me through the tears of my first dead patient and taught me the correct approach to the grieving family. 'You've been so kind doctor.'

'That's okay, I only filled out the blood forms,' you reply. 'Now hand over the chocolates, I've got cremation fees to collect.'

And we fell asleep in front of the telly among the discarded coffee cups and cigarettes, lovingly, in each other's arms. Well, almost.

Half an hour later I was bleeped back into consciousness with a call to the haematology ward, to stick a drip line in some kid who was having a blood transfusion. Haematology wards are full of people who get transfused their whole lives, and their veins are fibrous and thrombosed by the time the nurses are calling people like me over to cannulate them.

This guy looked about twelve.

'Hi,' I said, trying to be chummy, since he was a kid. He looked up from his book like I was the butler. 'How old are you?' I asked, doing my best to knock up a slightly dishevelled bit of early-morning bedside friendliness.

'I'm thirty-one, you prick. It's thalassaemia. It makes me look younger.' Fabulous. 'You'd better get this in first time, you know. The nurses have already fucked up my left arm.' I smiled: which is what you'd do. 'Jesus Christ,' he sighed, and turned back to his book.

I opened up the shrink-wrapped bits of kit I needed to stick a line into his nasty little veins, thinking about (in order): how nice it would be to get back into bed; how amazing it was that I had managed to qualify knowing so little haematology; and how cool it would be if you could buy some kind of magic beam that would morph shitty patients into beatific angels on sight.

So his comment 'That nurse has got fabulous tits' felt like a bit of a turning-point in our doctor–patient relationship. I looked up, grinning, but held fast to neutral territory.

'I wouldn't know about that, sir,' I replied, reaching for my saline flush and feeling pretty good about getting the line in first time.

'I can't believe you called me "sir". You called me sir! You really think I'm thirty-one. You must know fuck all.' He laughed noisily in the direction of the nursing station to get their attention, with his eyes wide open. 'This doctor knows fuck all! He thinks I'm thirty-one! You fuckwit!'

The patients around us start waking up. I think about making a sharp exit or at least a sharp remark (or maybe just twatting him), but then remember I'm the doctor. I guess it must get pretty boring being a kid in a hospital.

A Wayward Needle

I've gone and got bloody AIDS. I'll be dead in ten years. I shall devote myself to working in a lab, desperately struggling to find a cure, which will tragically be developed just weeks after my painful, lingering demise. They will read out at my funeral my last wish, that the fruits of my work should be donated free to an African workers' HIV cooperative, so that others may live on after my pain is over.

I've got bloody AIDS.

By which I mean, of course, I've had a needlestick injury. Not just any old needlestick injury of course. The kind of needlestick injury where the donor (what a sweet turn of phrase) is a drug-using alcoholic with psychiatric problems. The kind of donor who is stacked to the gills with every risk factor you can bloody think of, the bastard bastard bastard!

Deep breath. First let me tell you what a good boy I was. I was wearing my rubber gloves. I mean, I may as well have been wearing black satin ballgloves up to my elbows for all the difference they made, but I was wearing them when that idiot flinched his arm, which moved his hand, which pushed my elbow against the cotsides, which stopped me lifting my hand clear, which held the hollow needle filled with murderous blood, which eased its way gently into my glove.

And when I pulled it off there was a needle-shaped hole in it and when I looked at the side of my thumb there it was! The teeniest little miniscule pinprick, quite possibly even the smallest dot of nothing at all that I have ever seen. I beheld it in awe: should I chop off my hand?

I rushed to show the nurse. 'I know I should be sensitive about this, doctor,' she said, 'but that's the crappiest littlest needlestick injury I've ever seen. In fact, that's not a needlestick injury. It didn't even go into your hand. That's not even where it hit.' She held up the glove for comparison.

What a cow. I had just contracted bloody AIDS and still I was getting bullied by nurses.

Clearly I needed to see a doctor. Top-notch medical cover is a perk in this job and on this occasion it came in the form of a rather famous A&E consultant. 'The drugs only really work if you take them within an hour,' he said.

'Fabulous,' I replied: it only happened ten minutes ago.

'Why don't you register at the front desk?' he said.

Sounds time-consuming, I thought. Who does he think I am: a patient?

'How about we just chop off my hand right away and then I can start on some intravenous AIDS drugs?'

Neither of us were laughing, so I wasted ten minutes trying to register in my own A&E department, desperately fighting off visions of lurid computer animations with hundreds of little HIV viruses all busily replicating in my bloodstream. A&E consultants are the hardest bastards in the world.

So we filled out the forms and he told me the risks and he took some blood for storage and finally I was allowed to get my hands on some ridiculously potent anti-retroviral drugs: three brown tubs of huge yellow horse-medicine tablets. And then I had to wait thirty-six hours for my SHO to nobly but gently convince our acutely delirious (and actually rather sweet) patient that we needed a confidential HIV test on him. The rules on things like consent are made by *Guardian*-reading do-gooders with Cultural Studies degrees on committees where everyone wears black polo-neck sweaters – and for a day and a half I was seriously considering switching teams and becoming a reactionary old bigot.

So let me tell you about the drug side-effects. I thought it was bad enough when I took too much aspirin for a hangover and it made my haemorrhoids bleed. These HIV drugs are monstrous: my heart heavy with the knowledge that I was over-reacting outrageously and that the drugs were almost certainly unnecessary, I struggled zombie-like to the toilet every half hour to release another payload of loose, green stool, post-on-call with twenty-three new patients on four hours' sleep, feeling like I was indulging in some morbid new brand of disease tourism to the land of HIV positivity. At least it kept my mind off thoughts of my own mortality.

So, obviously he was negative. It took me days to recover. And this is what I am thinking right now: it's not too late to get out of acute hospital medicine. Maybe I should bite the bullet, apply for some NHS-issue family doctor sideburns, buy a pair of corduroy trousers, and become a GP.

Surgical House Officer

Provincial, Boring and Uncool

Someone's pulled the grass out from under my feet: one moment I'm a medical house officer in a glamorous and well-funded central teaching hospital, the next I'm a skivvy for a bunch of surgeons in some district general hospital's concrete box in the middle of nowhere. How did this happen?

It's all part of a grand experiment to disorient and abuse junior doctors. Every six months they move you on to some new alien hospital, and to get full registration with the general medical council you have to do six months of surgery as well as six months of medicine, for one very simple reason: surgeons, who make up about 10 per cent of medical graduates, need a vast army of barely qualified medical skivvies to do their dirty work on the wards.

What do we know about doing surgery? Nothing. We are Santa's little helpers. As my new senior house officer pointed out on the first day of the job: 'I am the SHO. You are my 'ho.' He likes Eminem.

I hold retractors in theatre. I do bloods and cannulas. I write the results in the notes. I am barely still a doctor, apart from pre-op clinics.

'Do you have any allergies? No. Still got that hernia? Jolly good. Get your ECG over there. Next.'

With time the hypnotic repetition could become quite thera-peutic, a bit like knitting or raffia work. And as ever in medicine there is always scope for invigoratingly deathtastic cock-ups.

What I don't understand is why this all has to take place in a hospital in an anonymous little market town somewhere between twenty and sixty miles outside London. Let's call it Boreham General.

Like all the other district general hospitals I went to as a medical student, it was pretty easy to find. You just pitch up at

36

the right train station on your first day of work and aim for the big incinerator tower. At medical school we used to consider our brief sojourns to places like this as cautionary tales. 'I'd better concoct a pretty convincing CV before I qualify,' we would all secretly plot in the college library, 'because otherwise I'll end up working in Boreham General for the rest of my life, like all those other lost souls.'

So here I sit, staring blankly at the walls, in Bedside Manor, the small concrete bunker where they keep the junior doctors at night when they are not using them. I could go out with my new colleagues and drink to excess, once more, in the plastic pub around the corner. Or I could sit in my room and stare blankly at the walls. Some of the other HOs are old hands at district general life.

'Bedside Manor? This is a bloody palace, son,' they say in broad Yorkshire accents. 'When I were a lad, in Borebury General, the on-call doctor slept at t'bottom of t'sharps bin, snuggled up against t'used needles and empty glass vials, and we used to wash in t'dirty utility room on t'ward next to t'used colostomy bags.'

But don't let me knock the old place. Because for everything I might say, there is one thing about this hospital that left me utterly disorientated for days: everybody – and I mean everybody – is outrageously, absurdly, almost surreally friendly.

'Good morning doctor,' they chirp.

'Hi . . .' I replied for the first few days, trying not to look suspicious. This is not what it was like when I was working for Prof in a teaching hospital.

But it's real. This is the only hospital in the town. The patients do not routinely abuse you. The little old lady in the Friends hospital shop, which still sells Curly Wurlys for 'seventeen pence please, dear', we know each other by name. Her shop is not a prefabricated corporate franchise on a unit of glisteningly valuable retail space in a busy hospital foyer. To be honest, it looks like she built it herself one quiet weekend in 1972.

And last night we all went out with the nurses to the local out-of-town entertainment multiplex centre, with its seven-screen cinema and three restaurant-bar-nightclub venues, for the fortnightly '999' night. ('Where the emergency services let their hoses out.') I never saw ward sisters in their mid-forties get drunk like that in my old hospital.

Who cares about the art galleries and concerts I was always too tired to make it to in my old job? Who cares if everyone over the age of nineteen is married around here? Who cares if surgical ward rounds start at 7.45 in the morning? At least they're over by nine. If I were twenty years older and my social life had been neatly cauterized by a collection of small children, I might seriously consider bringing them up somewhere not entirely unlike this shithole.

Grappling with Racism

'I don't trust that Paki much.'

I always find comments like this a little bit tricky to deal with. When a patient (who in this case was in a fairly bad way) focuses such forthright racism on a senior colleague, you're trapped between too many conflicting values and motivations. One fairly compelling option is to look them square in the eye, index finger raised aloft, and suggest plainly: 'Why don't you stop being such a racist twat?'

It's a strategy with obvious flaws. I want to be the patient's friend, I want him to trust me and help me get him better. I don't want to alienate him on first sight. And it seems likely that his comment was conceived, on some weird level, to be part of a Caucasian bonding moment, by someone confronting mortality more than a little bit sooner than they had planned, and who felt scared and alone and surrounded by strangers.

Is it necessarily my job to go around challenging the unacceptable values of every person I encounter in the workplace?

Even if I thought I was doing work for the public good? I am, in fact, the only Caucasian doctor on our firm, and also by far the most junior.

'You're awlright, mate. I know I can trust you. It's just that lot that bother me.' He smiles warmly. I start to fumble with embarrassment.

'Well, really it's all, no, right, OK, shit,' I offer, looking at the floor. You're an idiot and you are definitely trusting the wrong man, I think to myself. I consented a patient for the wrong operation last week (although he had the right one). Perhaps this is karma in action.

I struggle to work out which of our team it is whose appearance has so offended him. They are all male (there are no women in surgery), they all went to public school in the United Kingdom, and his terminology didn't seem to fit with any of the West African, Arabic and Oriental genes on our firm.

Either way, in five hours' time all three of them were going to be up to their elbows in racist abdomen. Do I tell my bosses what he said about them? And if so, should I tell them before or after they get their scalpels out? The temptation is great.

In the end I belly out and decide not to mention it at all. Does this make me a conspirator? The patient seemed to think so.

'I'd like a bit of that,' he said to me that afternoon on his way back from theatre in the lift, pointing at a physiotherapist's perfect bubble butt. 'Know what I mean, eh doc?' he continued, as if I were his best mate. Everyone else in the lift stared at me in astonishment.

This, I should point out, is the only interesting thing that has happened to me in three weeks. Apart from the novelty of having patients under the age of seventy, being a surgical house officer is so tedious that on some afternoons I have almost gnawed my own leg off with boredom, and the only relief comes when I am on-call and get to see fresh patients in A&E.

The basic problem with surgery is that unless you're into the railway modelling aspect of it all, it's a bit of a one-laugh gag. I can still remember the first time I went to theatre as a medical student, being amazed at how counter-intuitive it was to stick a knife into somebody's guts: it was all I could do to stop myself reaching out and grabbing the surgeon's hand as it zoomed in on the patient's tummy and shouting 'Are you mad? You were going to cut that bloke's tummy open with that knife! Somebody call the police!'

Now I just stand there holding a retractor while they talk about sport and tits – like I said, there are no women in surgery – or discuss new and exciting surgical tools, just like the DIY nerds that deep down they know they really are.

And in the morning we do 8 a.m. ward rounds on twenty patients in half an hour, during which I don't have time to find the notes for each patient, let alone write in them. Then they all bugger off to theatre while I have a little paperwork party all on my own. In my medical job I was rushed off my feet, because pressure of work (and the loveliness of my team) meant that I actually helped work out how to get patients better, as well as sorting through the administrative tedium.

But I spend most of my day here twiddling my thumbs, with the unnerving feeling that there must be something I should be doing and that it probably involves standing up in theatre holding a retractor for four hours, wearing blue pyjamas and a silly hat.

A Serious Case of Surgeon's Penis

I have been reduced to hiding patients from my consultant. You try telling him that the little old lady whose gall bladder he has whipped out can't go home, just because some occupational therapist says she can't make a cup of tea safely in the practice kitchen.

'Out!' he shouts (and he does really shout it) waving his arms around at head height, then moves on to the next patient.

Now naturally I assumed that this was nothing more than rather camp affectation on his part: but the same afternoon, the sister on ward 6B bleeps to let me know she has 'sorted out' Mrs Henderson.

'You know how upset John can get,' she says, referring to our consultant surgeon (whose name is Mr Cobb and definitely not John) as if she were his devoted and long-suffering wife.

The next morning the patient has in fact disappeared. Until the nurses on 3C, an orthopaedic ward, bleep me after lunchtime.

'When are you coming to see your patient, then?' (I don't know if you could hear the silent 'you bastard' on the end of that sentence). Sitting in the corner is dear old Mrs Henderson, and she still doesn't have a clue where she is. Neither does my consultant: as far as he is concerned, she's back festering in sheltered accommodation. After the mess he made of her insides, I was amazed she even woke up, but there it is. Don't tell anyone, for God's sake.

The patients who have been around for a while think this is all very entertaining. Mr Parkett has been moored to the ward by his ropey waterworks since before I arrived. He has been having secret rendezvous with Mrs Henderson in the smoking room, and now knows that I, too, have secret liaisons with her at the end of every ward round.

Unfortunately, I'm not allowed to chat with him like I used to, because he has offended sister. Deluded, perhaps, by the sheer volume of attention that has been lavished on his penis and the central role it has come to play in his life, he has taken to wearing it outside his trousers (sometimes he just wears anti-blood-clot stockings up to his thighs his dressing gown open rather louchely as he sits out in his chair).

'I'm not going to talk to you until you put your penis away, Mr Parkett,' I say with a broad smile, on sister's instructions, and he rolls his eyes.

So, as you can see, I'm on the wards all day and I'm bored. All the action in surgery happens in outpatients (which is fairly

41

boring) or theatre (which is very boring). All I do all day is paperwork and drip lines. I'm bored of being boring by boring on about it, nobody ever teaches me anything and even bum jokes aren't funny any more.

I spent the whole of yesterday morning with my eye on a lens attached to a pipe up someone's arse, inflating their colon with air from a pump to get a good view, and replenishing it as it blew out of the margins of their anus, occasionally with such force that I could feel its cool wind against my nose. It wasn't funny. It wasn't even gross. I can have tea and cake in an atmosphere misty with bowel gas without even a twitch. But it is very, very boring.

The only interesting thing about my job is when I get to witness the ball-breaking insensitivity of surgeons.

'Your toes!' they start to shout, as we walk up to the foot of a bed.

'Yes, doctor?' replies a little old lady in a floral nightie who, as far as she was concerned, had only popped in to show her GP her cold painful feet out of passing interest. 'They'll probably drop off by themselves in the next week or so.'

And then we rush away to finish the ward round by nine, so that everyone can get to theatre.

But let's go back to that little old lady, because those fourteen words were literally all he said to her.

'Did I catch that right?' she must be thinking. 'Did that bloke just tell me my feet are going to fall off? He didn't seem to be making much of an issue out of it. Perhaps I misunderstood.'

And worst of all, that brashness, that hurried I've-got-some-thing-terribly-important-to-do-with-a-big-knife-over-there stride, is starting to rub off on me. The other day I was a little bit rude to a nurse, albeit a nurse who bleeped me three times in half an hour to write up some non-urgent fluids that she then didn't even bother to put up.

But in medicine you must never forget your place. In medi-cine the hierarchy is even worse than the military, and the nurses love it: they love having a little junior doctor they can bully and they think it's so cute when the little baby house officers try to get angry.

'I'm not going to talk to you until you put your penis away, Dr Foxton.'

And so, rather delightfully, a new ward catchphrase is born.

Foxton Triple Therapy

Surgery is like one big pyjama party. I was woken at 7.55 by Clara – a surgical house officer I find rather dishy – bouncing up and down on my bed in the on-call doctor's room and shouting 'Wakey-wakey, Dr Sleepyhead! Your ward round awaits!'

After a routine check that my genitals have not fallen out of the front of my theatre blues (a hazard of using them as pyjamas) I spring up and pull on a white coat for the morning round.

You cannot begin to imagine the pain and misery of a night on-call, followed by a day at work. If you could, you probably wouldn't all keep coming in at 3 a.m. with that bit of tummy ache that has been troubling you for six months. I have to say, on the whole, I am not very impressed with your pain threshold; not to mention your common sense.

Go back to bed, I am tempted to write in the notes as my clinical plan, *and leave me alone to sleep*. But that's not what they want: they want hospital lights and hospital beds and hospital hysteria.

'Ooh, I was up at that hospital the other night,' you can hear them saying, after being sent packing the following morning. 'Accident and Emergency it was. They had me on one of them drips and everything. They still never found out what it was.'

Yes we did. You had tummy ache. Now go to bed and be good.

It breaks my heart to say it, but you know for sure that they wouldn't do it if it wasn't free of charge. Still, at least in this job we get a cosy on-call room on a staircase near the wards. In my last job we had to sprint a hundred yards across open gangland territory in central London at 3 a.m. when the cardiac arrest bleep went off.

And, of course, now I've got this new job, now I'm a surgeon, I don't have to do too much thinking, because you only ever see the same five things over and over and over again and because thinking isn't butch enough for surgeons. Surgeons stand in theatre looking hard and calling their house officers 'big girls' for not being able to hold retractors for hours on end. They don't like to think. It makes their willies hurt.

So, after I flourished my sleepy way through the new admissions (two lots of appendicitis, one sub-acute obstruction, and three crap tummy aches), we stumbled across a patient from the wards whom I had seen, who was 'short of breath' and coughing up goo overnight.

Needless to say, without a moment's thought I instituted the patented Foxton Triple Therapy for chest symptoms: antibiotics in case it's an infection, diuretics in case it's heart failure, and a salbutamol nebulizer, partly on the off-chance that she had a bit of chronic lung disease and partly because those big see-through masks with clouds of mist coming out of them look fabulously pneumatic and Victorian and it's an aesthetic our elderly patients often seem to appreciate.

The registrar was not impressed. Deciding for the first time in his life to take an interest in the medical management of our surgical patients, he held his hand aloft theatrically. I could sense a rare moment of loquacity coming on.

'It is as if,' he said, with a grandiose smile, 'you had walked into a darkened room filled with flies, and started firing off rounds from a machine-gun at the walls.'

We all peered at the silver pan of poo that the nurse had brought for us. It contained a puddle of green-and-red semi-formed stool, which smelled metallic and vegetal in the way that only antibiotic-induced pseudomembranous colitis does. I was definitely not guilty: she had only been on the drugs for twelve hours.

'Well done, doctor. And with which ten drugs will you be attacking her bowel to reverse the effect?'

The Evil Sister on Ward 7B stared at me. I froze, immobilized by the injustice of it all and the complex damage limitation analysis running through my brain. Should I mention that it was *his* twelve days of cefuroxime and metronidazole that had trashed her bowels?

'Blink if you can hear me, Dr Foxton.'

Clearly not. Should I chance a matey comment to defuse the atmosphere? Something implicitly sexist, perhaps? They seem to like those ones.

He walked over and put his mouth menacingly close to my ear.

Shit, I thought, he's going to bite my fucking ear off. He smiled and whispered into it: 'You're obviously mistaking me for someone who gives a shit, Dr Foxton. She's been incontinent and doolally in a nursing home for six years. I can't believe you even got out of bed for her.' He returned to his usual bark. 'Right. Well done. I'm going to theatre.'

And I was alone once more.

A Cheering Parsnip

Being your doctor is worse than being your mum. Unconditional love, that's what you expect. You think your mortality is so bloody important that we're weird if we ever want to go home.

'Doctor, exactly why hasn't my mother had a normal bowel movement since this morning?'

'I'm not going home until I get the result of my scan.'

Oh yes you are, honey.

Fortunately, the unreasonable bad behaviour of the unappeasable few has allowed me to develop a professional emotional distance. I have been watching, and it has happened to all of us.

We are cleaved from the reality of your pain. Those moments when the nurses bleeped to tell us that Mr P.'s family were here again, demanding to see a doctor (about why being fat and eating shit your whole life gives you bowel cancer, perhaps) and making ludicrous grunting noises about going to the Press and the General Medical Council: we shan't be staying late for you any more. Thank you, and bad luck.

Fortunately, people are still sticking interesting things up their bottoms to keep us all in good spirits. I am called from my bleary sleep at 3 a.m. and curse my way across the barren snow-cursed wasteland that separates my room from the hospital, to find as I wake on arrival that I am wearing theatre bottoms, a white coat, an orange scarf, a woolly hat and a medical school t-shirt with the phrase DISEASES ARE AFRAID OF ME scribbled across the front.

Nights on-call are so weird you sometimes wonder if they ever happened at all. Did I really wake up at 3 a.m. when my bleep went off, and spend twenty minutes heroically (and single-handedly) managing a torrential gastrointestinal bleed before retiring once more to bed? I sometimes wonder. Or did I merely answer the phone, mumble some reassuring sleep-fudge to the nurse, go back to sleep, and dream the entire episode? If so, did the patient die? And will I be arrested?

Anyway, it's not every day that you get called to see a patient with a parsnip lodged in their anus. Root vegetables in general are pretty popular, apparently, but don't let me get away with being sage about it: this was my first vegetable-in-arse call. I was delighted, but my professionalism was breathtaking.

Now, for the purposes of this anecdote, there are certain things you have to know about surgeons. For historical reasons their hobbies are sport, sexism, and homophobia, and although there are almost certainly some female surgeons somewhere I've never seen one. An example of surgeons in action: if I am not able to hold a retractor for long enough in theatre, this is because I am either a 'poofter' or a 'big fat girl'.

Outraged? I suppose they don't mean any harm. They're just

over-qualified manual labourers with aspirations to working-class chic, after all, but they all went to public school so every now and then they're going to get the tone a bit wrong. They think they're big and clever. So what if they're doctors? I'm too tired to think about it.

Anyway, this patient has a parsnip up his arse – I can't even be bothered to share his explanation for how this might have happened – and we have to retrieve it.

God knows why he can't shit it out. But there you go, I'm just a house officer, I'm as much in the dark as you are on most of this medical stuff. Needless to say, I call for senior assistance. First the SHO tries his hand, but every time he thinks he's caught it, the tapered end slips further in. Then we think about instruments, but the registrar is worried about perforating the bowel. There is only one option: we sit on it.

In theatre next morning we find our patient once more on his side, this time lightly anaesthetized. Apparently, there is a scene out there for using ketamine as an aid to fisting, the anaesthetist tells me. I pretend not to know what either of those things are, because I'm too tired to cope with a weird conversation. Everyone gets down to business.

The SHO successfully grasps the misplaced vegetable through the grossly dilated anal orifice and begins to edge back. The tension in the room is almost unbearable. All eyes are upon him and, as he gently eases out the offending vegetable, success seems imminent. Suddenly, as it clears the anal verge, the patient's flaccid penis begins to twitch, and emits a steady stream of sticky grey fluid. No one can realistically deny it is semen.

Everyone turns to the SHO and the SHO turns to the registrar looking concerned. The registrar holds his index finger aloft and raises an eyebrow: clearly this is the most urgent moment of his entire homophobic sparring career. He is genuinely inquisitive.

'Charles, darling,' he smiles. 'Does that make you gay?'

Mrs G.'s Varicose Veins

Surgeons are far from being the intellectuals of the medical world.

'It's funny, surgery,' I said to my senior house officer one day. 'Sometimes it almost seems too straightforward: you know, someone has a bit of cancer in their bowel, we chop it out and stick the ends together; someone has a gammy leg with blocked blood vessels, so we chop it off and make a stump.'

He looks at me, baffled, scraping his knuckles along the corridor floor as we walk towards the endoscopy department.

'That's exactly what we do,' he says. We walk past the physiotherapist I've been unsuccessfully flirting with for three months. 'Right. Now I need you to book an urgent rigid bell-endoscopy for that physio, and I'll see you in theatre in five minutes.'

Dear God, not the operating theatre. Four hours of holding a retractor while the consultant points out a few bits of gristle, claiming they represent some anatomical structure I've forgotten ever existed. The worst of it all is that now, after three months in the job, they keep trying to involve me in the chopping side of things.

'Closer to the vein, follow the vein, dissect it out with the scissors – closer, don't be such a girl.'

Christ, I think, have you seen the size of that thing? It's a huge pipe full of blood and all your shouting is giving me the shakes. This could get messy.

'Come on, come on, we're going to cut it out anyway – she's got bloody varicose veins you fool, just dissect it down and make sure there's nothing funny going on.'

There is nothing funny going on.

'Right, now clamp it, open the fucker up and stick this vein stripper down the hole.'

I glance up as he passes me what looks like a bit of straightened-out coat-hanger.

There are times – when the mood takes him – that my consultant will try to make the work of a surgeon sound technical and sophisticated. I'm sure it's not just pretence. I'm sure they really do need an extensive lexicon of technical terms to describe what are undeniably very dextrous and careful manœuvres.

'Come on, come on, stick it down and wiggle it around! You're stripping the veins off, not catheterizing your boyfriend! Bloody get on with it!'

The vein starts to give a bit more and I pull it back gingerly. It makes a sound like poppers opening in quick succession on the back of a dress, as each connecting tributary gives way. My surgical mask hides the expression of disgust that crosses my mouth as I feel the vein popping a few millimetres looser with each tug, and ease it out. I work on the perforators with the funny little hook they use, poking it into the holes my SHO impatiently pokes with a pointed blade, and rooting around to see if I can pull out a stringy, bogey-like vein. It's actually rather satisfying and a lot like picking your nose: I find myself more and more absorbed in the process as I clean out dear old Mrs G.'s nasty varicose veins.

And then, to my horror, I realize that I have been conned into doing an operation.

And I feel pretty good about it. OK, this poor woman's legs are in a right old state, but she's just had surgery and that's just the way it is. I start to wash off the blood, quietly feeling rather professional as I sweep the brown antiseptic swab over her bloody calves. It all seems pretty damn good to me, and I look up hoping to catch my consultant smirking proudly. But he has run off to whine about hospital management in the coffee room, and there is just me and the SHO, who is quietly staring at the anaesthetist's breasts rising and falling as she reads the newspaper.

Needless to say, I feel rather big and clever about the whole episode, until I watch *Mad Max* on telly in the mess in the afternoon. I realize that whereas I might be pretty good at filling in forms and dishing out antiobiotics (and after nine months in the game I have to say I'm pretty damn good at it), and even if I can do varicose veins all by myself with a coat-hanger, one thing is certain: in a post-holocaust, urban-warrior situation after the revolution comes, when western society as we know it is in a state of terminal disarray and my insurgent revolutionary chums and me are hiding out in the foothills of some mountain range and they look at me as if I have the first clue what to do about our walking wounded, I'd still be worse than useless.

Barking Patients

Ten months of being a doctor and still nobody has put me in their will to spite their children. Instead, I am called to the ward at 3 a.m. (it's always 3 fucking a.m.) to see a patient who is throwing things at the nurses and barking in a high-pitched voice.

'I know that's usually your job, doctor, which is why I called you. Is he a friend of yours?'

She's cheeky, and my God she's beautiful.

Only five hours ago this man was a cheerful problem drinker with acute pancreatitis in casualty. What the fuck had the nurses done to him? I bleep the night nurse for a bit of back-up.

'You're the one who is paid all that money,' he chirps, 'so you're the one who is responsible for the patients.' He puts the phone down laughing.

Now, this is a baffling response, but not entirely unusual: often in a hospital, non-medical staff get a bit confused and start thinking that because doctors take responsibility for all the medical decision-making, they are also the only people who need to take any responsibility for anything at all. Under this tra-dition, anything that everyone else refuses to do on grounds of workload or taste becomes the job of the house officer: that'll be me, over here with the seventy-hour week.

I only wanted a bit of a hand, I think, feeling hurt. So what if I am white and over-privileged and sound a bit posh on the phone?

I decide to have a look at the guy. He throws an NHS water jug at the door and it hits me in the chest. I duck out again.

'Why don't you just sedate him?'

They all look at me. Normally, I'm a modern, liberal type who thinks we should all be able to sort out most problems of this nature with a bit of even-handed counselling. But there was no way this guy was going to let me close enough to find out how they'd made him bark like a dog, and he had just hit me in the chest with a full water jug, and I did now look as if I'd wet myself, and the overall picture was beginning to seriously impact on my gravitas in front of the sexiest nurse in the hospital.

'Give him four milligrams of midazolam would you, please, nurse?' I smile.

'Fuck off,' she suggests.

Briefly my mind flashes with the words 'incident form'. Doctors don't fill them out too much, because we're not creeps, but the nurses – we believe – are constantly relaying our every move back to the clinical incident Nazis.

'You try and give it,' she continues, with a broad smile on her face. This is worse than the day I lost my lucky Viagra promotional biro.

We walk over to the edge of the cubicle.

'Mr Bundy?' I call out, reassuringly.

An apple bounces off the door and he starts barking again. A reasonable man would have called security. A reasonable hospital would have had security staff.

A healthcare assistant holds out a motorcycle helmet.

'I can't wear that,' I say. 'I'm a doctor.'

She looks at me as if I just said it to show off in the pub. I ignore her and think through the options: body armour might help me survive the hostile environment of his side-room, but there was still no way I was going to get the drugs into his arm. My pocket textbook – usually so helpful – only suggested giving the drugs rectally. This seemed like it might further inflame an already difficult situation.

I walk in, bravely shielding my face and abdomen with my only two forearms: he is half sat-up in bed and struggling away at the small portable telly next to him, trying to remove it from the flimsy bracket mounting. I reckon I've got about thirty seconds to complete the operation before he manages to break it off and chuck it at my head.

He picks a banana from the bowl of fruit he has been keeping menacingly on his lap, but throws it aimlessly at the ceiling. I scan the room further and notice the umbrella near his right hand: and then I see the drip stand. I ease forwards and grab the litre bag of normal saline from its hook, retreating rapidly to below his line of sight at the foot of the bed.

I am James Bond, I think to myself as I crouch on the floor and inject the midazolam into the drip tube that is connected to his vein six feet away and start squeezing on the bag, imagining I can actually see its reassuring little benzodiazepiney molecules moving along the tube towards his arm. An apple slams into the wall behind me.

'Fucker!' he cries, with less enthusiasm. I squeeze harder on the bag, willing the fluid uphill and into his arm, feeling only marginally shielded by my white coat.

'Fff-fuc . . .'

And lo, he was tranquil.

A Game of Snap

I just want a job where I don't have to deal with penises all day – I'm thinking mainly of other surgeons.

'Blimey, did you see the state of that bloke's missus?'

My SHO was referring, in his most contrived working-class

tones, to the scantily clad and sheepish-looking partner of our new star urology patient.

'I'm not surprised he snapped his knob.'

Penis fractures, I should reassure you, are something of a rarity, hence our childlike excitement. A hardy perennial in medical student paranoias, you would know it if it happened to you: a sudden onset of tearing pain, immense swelling, terrifying bruising and, most strikingly, a very loud snapping sound.

The GP who referred the patient over the phone immediately had me down as just the kind of doctor-impostor beloved by the tabloids. It was 10 p.m. when I took the call, but I was still wrestling with a biblical hangover from the drug dinner the night before, and the moment my intuitively work-shy brain heard the word 'fracture', whole banks of on-call survival circuits flipped into action.

'I'll stop you right there,' I said, distractedly signing some blood results at the nursing station. 'Fractures go to the orthopods.'

'This man's fractured his boner, you cock. He needs an urgent urology opinion.'

I'd never heard a GP talk like that before: usually they're all sideburns and antidepressants. He'll be waiting until morning if I know the urologists, I think to myself.

'He's shitting his pants.'

And suddenly the immense gravitas of the situation came crashing down around my ears. Of course he is, I thought. Of course he's shitting his pants: he's just heard his willy snap in half.

'Right, let's have a look at the old chap then,' I said, trying to make the whole affair sound as innocuous as a nineteenth-century condom fitting.

It was a classic history: a little something to drink, she was on top, they got carried away; she was bearing down on him, he felt the old feller strain and bend, and retreated intuitively – but there was no give in the mattress, no room for manœuvre, no escape. Something had to go. And then – *snap!* Can you even begin to imagine?

Now, if there is one thing that medicine has taught me, it is an ability to suppress the urge to giggle, burst into tears or retch in any social circumstance. I reckon I'm pretty good at it. I can happily eat a lunchtime sandwich in a room full of open colostomies. In our daily rounds of manipulation and deceit, we constantly shimmy around the issues and tell porky pies, at least until the diagnosis is definite – all for your own good. In fact, I can't keep up the charade: we constantly lie to you, for our own convenience and amusement. At least, that's what most of you seem to believe. But I digress.

Christ, I'm bitter.

Although our urology consultant pulled a stroke of communication skills genius in outpatients last week, with the assistance of two young female medical students.

'I'd like you to examine this man's testicles for me, please,' he said, in his campest, most intimidating tones.

The two women obliged, intently palpating the twenty-year-old patient's testes.

'Well?' he barked.

'Two normal testes,' they both replied anxiously.

'Well, that's not bad, is it?' he roared. 'Two nice attractive young girls telling you that your balls feel normal. Plastic. Put them in myself six weeks ago. Bloody great big scar up to his arsehole.'

They were mortified, but the patient was beaming; and that is how it should be. We are mere tools for your emotional well-being.

Anyway, I gently opened out the trousers around this famous fractured penis and exposed, to my horror, a swollen, blue, mis-shapen, appalling, unpenislike blob.

Christ, I thought.

'Right,' I said, confidently.

And what happened next is the only saving grace of surgery,

a corner of medicine populated exclusively by sporty philistines and intellectual peasants with pretend working-class accents, questionable social values, and boringly glamorous girlfriends. What happened next was this: I phoned the registrar, the registrar phoned the consultant, the consultant came in from home at midnight and within an hour this poor man's willy was fixed and everyone except me had gone to bed happy.

And it was all free of charge.

Sex and the Single Doctor

When did my patients become the enemy? Apparently I'm a sex pest.

'I can't believe you were about to examine that woman without a chaperone.'

My registrar has a strong sense of self-preservation, and rightly so in the litigious environment of our pleasant little country hospital, where lawyers are rich and doctors come cheap, and the patients are never too shy to share their feelings with both.

The only time I ever even thought about getting a chaperone was when I was dealing with a seventeen-year-old appendix patient wearing a child-size T-shirt with FUCK ME BABY written across her breasts. Even then, the nurses made a huge fuss about how busy they were.

'I need a chaperone,' I said.

They looked at me wearily. 'We're very busy. Can't you just get on with it?'

I thought through being grumpy and decided to try and explain.

'The thing is, she's got FUCK ME BABY written all over her tits.'

Eyebrows were raised. That's the problem with chaperones: they raise the whole horrid issue and stick it right in your face.

I can't get over it. Telling a patient 'I'll just pop and get a chaperone' always seems to imply 'There's a reasonable possibility I'm a pervert.'

Which is weird, because I cannot even begin to tell you how asexual the environment of a hospital is, especially when you're sticking your finger in a businesslike fashion into your seventh anus of the afternoon. My finger still smells of poo afterwards – even through the rubber gloves. It is not sexy. It's just something I have to do, because who knows what manner of awful tumour or other nastiness you might have hidden up there.

'If you don't put your finger in it, you'll put your foot in it,' as my consultant says. And there's no way I'm putting my foot in it.

So, anyway, I tramped about the A&E department for a few minutes and eventually found myself a lovely overworked nurse to come and stand in the room, looking bored and embarrassed with me, while I lifted this utterly bemused fifty-year-old woman's breasts out of the way of her heart to stick my stethoscope on her ribcage, and we all quietly thought to ourselves about how times had changed and what a sad world we live in, or maybe I just think about things too much now that I've got a fifteen-shots-a-day coffee habit.

God knows how I thought I was going to hear anything anyway. My stethoscope's got a lot quieter since I dropped it into the bowl while bending over in the loo, and I don't know where to buy pipe-cleaners around here.

To get back to the whole sex thing, which is animating me painfully at the moment: I thought that, what with me being a dashing young doctor type these days, at the very least I was supposed to have a glamorous girlfriend.

Not a sniff.

Just because I have no time to myself and all I do outside of work is moan doesn't mean I'm not a nice person. And, boy, do I moan.

House officers exist only because hospitals are organizational disaster zones.

'Just go and chase the result of that scan will you, Michael?'

Unless I'm on-call – seeing patients in casualty – that is my whole day's work. Why do I have to tramp about chasing the bloody scan result? What's so difficult about it just coming up to the ward when it's done? It's not that I'm a snob about donkey work, but maybe you lot would be a bit less offensive to us if we spent our time helping to plough through the waiting lists in outpatients instead of being hospital porters. And I haven't had a girlfriend for a year.

'Nobody should have a girlfriend when they're a house officer,' says my registrar, who is keen to assert his butchness at every opportunity. 'You should just be shagging everyone in sight.'

Well, the nurses are all either over forty or think we're stuck-up middle-class brats; no one from the real world would touch us with somebody else's barge pole (quite right too); and the occupational therapists, social workers, and physios all think we're unfeeling bullies who don't care about the holistic picture and can't think about anything outside of our textbooks. Absolutely.

So now, get Mrs Bentley home before she catches that antibiotic-resistant pneumonia off the woman in the bed next door and dies, please, while I go and drink myself to death.

Physicians on Film

I don't know what's wrong with you lot, but if you want doctors to deal with your problems I suggest you stop treating us like a bunch of bastards.

I walked into a cubicle on the ward yesterday with my biggest, most beaming and helpful smile on my face (apparently there's a physiotherapist on the fifth floor who wants to snog me) to be met with a crowd of thugs and a video camera shoved up my nose.

Shit, I thought. An ambush!

'Right, so you're this doctor, are you?' said one thug. I looked down: white coat and a stethoscope. The cameraman pulled back to get a better view. 'Well, frankly, we're sick of this.'

Me too. Does that mean I can go to bed now?

'I'm terribly sorry. Is there a problem?' I frown, and think back to the communication skills classes of my misspent youth. I'm tolerant and charming. And terribly dishy. I am Dirk Bogarde in *Doctor in the House*.

'You're obviously completely fucking clueless and none of you know what's going on with my mother.'

Weirdly, for once, this wasn't true. His mother had diverticulitis, which is both easy and boring, and had developed it quite predictably at the end of a lifetime spent sitting on her fat arse eating bad food with no roughage and neglectfully raising a small village of thuggish offspring. She'd only been in hospital for about a day and she was already practically better, although still too fat to really walk.

So I settled down and gave them a frankly undeserved and rather fabulous five-minute package on diverticulitis: how you diagnose it, the best treatment, the most likely outcome . . . I even missed out the bit about how it was all her own fault and maybe they could all just hurry up and die of stupidity so I could get on with the rest of my job.

And I did it because normally I'm just a nice guy with a lot of sympathy and respect for other people, and not because I had a video camera shoved in my face. Actually, I rather enjoyed the video camera bit. It made me feel like one of those ropey media doctor types on telly, and secretly I've always rather fancied myself on *Richard and Judy*. I got well into my stride; I felt good about myself. I had put aside other commitments, put in some time and pacified the loons.

'Well, she didn't have that diverticulitis before she came into your hospital, did she?'

He was victorious. It's an interesting philosophical point, obviously: I guess until we said she had it, on some very weird and deep level, she didn't have diverticulitis. It was indeed my fault that his mother was ill. They zoomed in on my name badge again.

Unfortunately, you see, people have funny ideas concerning the abiding importance of their own mortality (believe me, it's very humdrum), and even more peculiar ideas about how the state is going to nobly tend to their needs, even though they have consistently voted to have it dismantled for the past two decades, just because they pay some paltry sum in taxes that wouldn't buy you a quick catheterization in any other country's health service.

Now, as a little baby house officer and, at least still in public, a nice guy, I don't feel I have the right to put these nasty, rude little people in their place. As a doctor you're supposed to not just cope with extreme-sports social interaction, but to manipulate it to everyone's mutual benefit. We had long and farcical communication skills practical classes at medical school specifically to train us up for it.

But last week I was blessed with a locum registrar – and temps, as everyone knows, neither give a shit nor take any. So when I dragged him in to cast a quick eye over another patient in A&E as a favour (before I had really given them a full workup), and we were met with 'When am I going to see a fucking consultant?' and the usual 'Why doesn't anyone know what's going on in this fucking shithole?', followed by the diagnostic 'I know my rights,' he was kind enough to restructure the rules of engagement in the following fashion.

'Until tomorrow morning, sir, I am in effect the consultant, whereas you are a rude man with a slightly sore tummy who deserves nothing. This nervous soul on my left has been a surgical doctor for four months. He is now your only doctor. Goodbye.'

He snapped the curtains shut and left me in the cubicle.

Thanks a bundle. No community spirit, locums.

But when I left to fetch a drug chart he was standing outside, wearing an enormous smile and carrying two cans of fizzy pop.

'The moment he gives you any shit, Mike, just tell him to

fuck off. And I'll see you for a game of pool in ten minutes or you're fired.'

Rock on, brother.

The Private Ward

Private medicine makes me sick. It doesn't do the patients too much good either. Because, in general, while nurses on private wards are very good at showing you their cleavage while serving up house red with your Medallions de Veau, when it comes to doing anything vaguely medical they tend to fall flat on their perfectly manicured arses.

Usually we only have to tolerate the private ward when our consultant, rather time-consumingly, drags his troop of NHS minions up there at the end of the ward round, in order to make himself look more important than he already clearly is. But now – since they closed half of the beds in the main hospital and merrily sacked the regular staff – the NHS bed manager insists on sub-letting beds off the private wing, which as well as being vastly expensive is also miles away (often through torrential rain) from the rest of the hospital, and hence an immense pain in the arse for myself, the most junior member of the surgical team and therefore the organizational donkey of the outfit.

But the main problem, when you have a patient who is kicking off quite as badly as Mrs Wilson was yesterday, is that frankly I wouldn't trust the nurses on Princes Ward to look after my cat.

I tell Pippa, the rather glamorous medical SHO, about my sick punter on the private patients' wing

'Oh Christ, not that lot,' she rolls her eyes. 'I wouldn't let them look after my coat while I went for a shit. I'd bleep the bed manager and get her moved if I were you.' She pauses and looks at the size of my immense patient list. 'Unless she's definitely going to die anyway, of course, in which case you might as well leave her there . . .'

She smiles. Obviously neither of us has ever made that kind of decision and acted on it, although part of us wishes we had, because that would make us as enormously hard as the kind of battle-weary registrars who do it without thinking.

For example, only the hardened soul of a registrar can order a Hollywood call for a patient who, for local political reasons or oversight, is inappropriately marked down for resuscitation when they inevitably arrest; and a Hollywood call, in case you didn't know, is where everybody shows up to the cardiac arrest like they're on *ER*, panting dramatically and bouncing up and down on the patient's chest, not even pretending to give them an electric shock, and giving the greatest performance of their stage career until such time as it is politically appropriate to pronounce the patient dead to the family.

Don't pretend to be shocked: just be grateful we don't break your granny's ribs in the course of an inappropriate resuscitation because you watch too many unrealistic medical dramas on telly to believe us when we tell you on the ward round that resuscitation never ever (ever) works.

Often this kind of decision depends on your boss's personal investment in the case.

'Oh yeah,' the registrar says when I called him about Mrs Wilson. 'She's that cholecystectomy that Mr Flanner fucked up last week. Very embarrassing. Fit as a fiddle beforehand. Better get the old girl a bed on ITU to die in.'

Now, inevitably, when ITU turn up to see this kind of patient they can smell a rat, because ITU doctors are far from stupid.

'This patient's fucked,' they say, having rapidly assessed the situation, and then there follows an elaborate game of mutual denial and stake-raising, much like poker. Except in my case, discretion at 5 a.m. is utterly beyond me and seems especially pointless when the doctor admitting to ITU that evening is someone I was screamingly drunk with the night before. I can't lie with that kind of bond, particularly when it's less than twenty-four hours since he leant on my shoulder in the loos of some godforsaken smalltown nightclub and giggled, 'Can you believe I'm in charge of fucking ITU in five hours' time?'

So I call ITU.

'John,' I say, 'I've got this punter.'

He whinges.

'You're always full,' I say. 'Kick someone out. Cobb fucked up this lady's cholecystectomy. She's going to die. Can we have a bed on ITU please?'

He wants to know what for.

'So she can die in it, John. It probably won't take long. It's all very embarrassing, apparently. I don't understand these things. I'm just a house officer.'

But inside I know it: he's not going to give me the bed on ITU, and she's going to die, and she's going to do it slowly and grudgingly at 5 a.m. absolutely miles away in that ridiculous private wing. My legs will hurt, and the rain will mess up my new haircut.

Top Tips

I used to be a happy-go-lucky kind of person. But then, exactly one year ago today, I became a junior doctor: a house officer, a doormat, a sleepless, undead zombie, the whipping boy for impatient relatives and work-shy administrative staff. My registrar shouted at me, my patients died on me, my girlfriend left me, and everything was my fault.

Then I became a bastard.

But now it's all over and I'm sad to be moving on. It's a bit like those documentaries about kidnap and torture victims who finally get released and then decide they're in love with their tormenters. I'll miss the fizzy pop crisis meetings at 3 a.m. with the anaesthetist. I'll miss flirting with radiographers to get my patients' scans done. I'll miss rummaging through a huge folder of crap on the ward round and still not being able to find a good excuse for not having the blood results in there. Maybe I'll even miss the nurses bleeping me incessantly about pointless nonsense.

And I'll miss my friends, especially for the moments of utter hysteria on weekend ward cover, in the middle of the night, when I called my medical SHO for help, practically in tears, no food and no sleep, and presented him with three simultaneous patients all symptomatic with critically low blood pressures and all for no apparent reason. Both of us knew there were several far more fucked-up patients needing urgent attention at the other end of the hospital, and he whispered gently: 'For God's sake, just write up some fluids and run for your sanity, before they kill you.'

Maybe they were all lessons I needed to learn: because now I'm unflappable. Go on. Try and flap me.

Patient vomiting blood with a haemoglobin of six? You'll have to try harder than that.

A patient has found out from a cleaner in the ward that they've got cancer, plus a side order of furious relatives? I'll deal with it.

Horrible nurses calling you slack when you've been busting a gut with no sleep for what feels like a week? Well, we stopped caring what they think long ago.

So, as I pack up my few possessions and prepare to move out of Bedside Manor, the filthy concrete box where they store all the junior doctors at night, I wipe a delicate salty tear from my haggard eyes and prepare to write a handover list for the wide-eyed innocent young doctor, fresh from medical school, who will replace me.

But the patients are boring, irrelevant, smelly and whiny: the duty of a new doctor is to survive his first year intact, and one of the duties of an old lag is to help them through. So here are some words of advice for young people.

Rule One: DO NOT PISS ABOUT. You are a doctor. Do not swear on the wards: instead, comb your hair every morning and whistle hymns as you go about your day. Your geriatric patients will love you for it. Remember to swear about them behind their backs. It will make you feel better about their pain, and your colleagues will cherish you for it.

Rule Two: DO NOT PISS ABOUT. Do not go home on time leaving jobs undone, like everyone else who is not a doctor. You chose the job, now you pay the price. Always check the blood results. Keep perfect jobs lists and do them all, because for every ten things you forget one will reap disaster. And it will torture you for the rest of your days.

Rule Three: DO NOT PISS ABOUT. Get out of work as early as possible, while still obeying Rule Two. You are only contracted for sixty-four hours. Live your life. Grasp every opportunity to get drunk and have sexual intercourse with multiple casual partners.

Rule Four: BUY A BLOODY GREAT BIG FILE WITH LOADS OF POCKETS. Fill it with everything you need: blood forms, X-ray forms, pens, a pocket house officer survival guide and voodoo dolls of the nastiest nurse on each ward. It will save your life.

Rule Five: DO NOT EXPECT TO BE HAPPY. You will cry. You will hide in the toilets as the patients seem to drop like flies, and you will read your pocket textbook and you will weep. You will feel like you can't go on, more than you can ever possibly imagine, and you will want to die.

Rule Six: STOP BEING SUCH A PUSSY. I'm as clueless as you are. Just get on with it and I'll see you in the mess in half an hour.

Blood on a Greek Island

Astonishingly, I'm on holiday. Not that it makes any difference.

'Are you really a doctor?' asked the holiday rep in our cheesy hotel on the Greek island of Shaggos. I could see she was giving me the same look that all my elderly patients give me: a look that says 'You don't look a day over three years old; but if you say you're a doctor, I suppose I'll have to believe you.'

Hastily I parried with my earnest-but-friendly-doctor expression, trying at the same time to maintain a flirtatious smile, for

– as is traditional for holiday reps on the island of Shaggos – she was almost offensively attractive and, more importantly, she looked like she was about to furnish me with an opportunity to deploy my immense intellectual prowess, in a sensitive and crowd-pleasingly New-Mannish fashion.

'I've got an awful sore throat,' she frowned into the sunshine, emphasizing (astonishingly) her breasts as she stroked her neck. 'And I've got to do Strip Bingo in half an hour.'

'Gosh,' I gulped. Strip Bingo. I'd never had someone smoke a cigarette sensuously in front of me while complaining about their sore throat.

'Gargle with aspirin,' I suggested. There was no way I was going to tell her to give up smoking when she was clearly so good at it.

So you can well imagine what happened next. First I was approached at my sun-lounger by a young family (and if there's anything worse than youthful policemen, it's watching dads getting younger than you).

'My daughter,' began the man in his early twenties, brandishing a big stick in one hand and a small child in the other, 'has developed a strange rash on her fingers, from the fibreglass in this snooker cue.'

Cluelessness has been a recurrent theme in my medical career. Most things you can look up if you need to and, more specifically, I spent the whole dermatology course in bed with my girlfriend (dermat-holiday we called it). I smilingly admitted I was clueless and suggested avoiding the snooker cue in future, but they all gazed at me, worriedly – as if their faith in doctors, medicine, and all western rational and scientific belief systems was waning, because of me.

I back-pedalled, in the name of good public relations for the profession, and lamely suggested some weak steroid cream, if it didn't 'clear up later'. It was an act of shameless and witch-doctorish mystification, I know, but from what little I remember of the subject it was no lamer than what most dermatologists would have come up with under similar circumstances. And more importantly, I was beginning to prepare a short speech in my head: Look. You can ask me whatever you like, but since I'm on holiday, I'm allowed to be as stupid as I like, OK?

The sun sank in the sky and I lazily settled in for dinner by the poolside. Halfway through my meal I was presented with a weeping and infected sore in the middle of a huge Geordie shin, which had clearly been missing most of its skin for several days.

'I fucked my shin when I was pissed,' said the huge Geordie attached to the limb, as I took another mouthful of squid. 'Now it hurts like shit. Are youse really a doctor?'

Barely, I thought to myself, and suggested TCP, which only led to more disappointment. Christ. Am I your mother?

So, over the course of the next three days, my rather louche poolside clinic stretched to: a recurring case of gout; disfiguring acne; three banged knees; a bleeding nose; and some rather invigorating concussion that could quite easily have turned very nasty. I suspect (being a rather vain kind of person) that I might have enjoyed the whole thing if I'd had the first clue what to do with any of them, but medical school teaches you about heart attacks, freaky rheumatology drugs, and the microscopic appearance of vanishingly rare tumours of the willy. It does not teach you about banged knees.

So that's why, with the realization that both medical school and house jobs have left me useless as a doctor for proper everyday stuff, I am joining almost everyone else from my year of house officers and doing my first job as a senior house officer in A&E. And here I will deal with this kind of minor crap day in and day out, for six months, until such time as I am very competent and very bored.

In an ideal world, you probably wouldn't have your most inexperienced junior doctors working smack bang on the front line in A&E, seeing every punter out of the ambulance before they get handed over to the real professionals. But there it is: you try getting anyone else to do it.

Casualty

Land of the Absurd

Could those of you who are drunk please go home? And there are so many of you, scattered decoratively about the A&E department like a series of lovingly hand-tooled porcelain figures: *Drunk Person Receiving Stomach Pump*; *Drunk Person Counselling Wife after Unconvincing Suicide Attempt*; *Drunk Person Contemplating Mortality in a Bowl of Bloody Vomit*; and my personal favourite, *Drunk Person Covered in Pond Weed Who has Tossed a Boiling Casserole Down Himself while Wearing Y-fronts*.

I try not to wince as I tease apart yellow underpants from saggy burnt flesh (because I do still have feelings) and distract the patient by taking a quick history.

'Were you drunk?' I hazard.

He hangs his head, picking algae out of his chest hair. 'Yes,' he slurs, 'quite drunk.'

I nod, caringly. Burns mean nothing to me. If they go red, they just need clever dressings, and dressings are a mysterious world, understood only by nurses. If they go white and the patient loses sensation, then you're truly buggered and we refer on to people cleverer than us, who prune it out.

I carefully examine his willy: he seems to have got off quite lightly. The worst-case scenario for burnt peripheries is a circumferential burn and I was worried that by removing his underpants we might have degloved his old feller. But apparently, in a moment of drunken clarity, he had the presence of mind to run for the garden and jump in the pond.

Accident and emergency is the random anecdote generator of the NHS, the strange attractor to which all ridiculousness will gravitate. The worst possible outcome of every risk you ever took is prominently on display. In our weekly teaching sessions, they try to encourage us to take a history and think through the mechanism of the injury.

'So this girl was driving home in a mini,' says the registrar as he takes me over to a patient in the assessment bay. 'Drunk.' She is on a spinal board. 'Very old car, welded together by her boyfriend, the wheels flew off and the car skidded along on its floor.' He grabs hold of the blanket. 'We spoke to the firemen' – he takes on a conspiratorial air, preparing for the denouement like he's a character in an Agatha Christie whodunit – 'and they said the floor had been peeled back.' He is hugely pleased with his detective work, and triumphantly pulls back the blanket to reveal: no feet. 'Yes,' he beams, as the orthopaedic team arrives smelling of cigarettes, 'she wiped them off on the road.'

But the worst of it is the unbreathable stench of the street drinker. Now, I'm not an unfeeling man and on an objective level I have a great deal of sympathy with the way your lifestyle options can narrow down to a pretty unappealing margin. But I'm no saint and it's difficult to be right-on when you're exposed to the socially unacceptable edge of other people's fuck-ups. This, for example, is why we don't want the police making political decisions about tearaways and drug-users.

This man had a smell that seeped into my clothing. If you breathed through your mouth to avoid the smell you could taste him. The fact is, we can't go round dishing out scarce trolleys to people for a good night's sleep, because even if things do slow down at 3 a.m. there is a matter of principle at stake. Actually, because it's August, all the doctors in A&E are new and we all take twice as long as we should to see patients, so things don't really slow down at 3 a.m. anyway. This, you may have noticed, is why a few more punters than usual have died on trolleys after eighteen-hour waits over the past few weeks. They don't tell you that in the press releases.

Normally the nurses deal with booting out the nutters, but on this occasion even our bullish sister was getting nowhere. She called me over to see if the dread hand of my doctorly authority could sort out the situation.

'I'm afraid you have to go now,' I say.

The pissed punter sits up and mumbles something. I look at Sister enquiringly.

'He says he loves you. You're his best mate,' she explains.

'That's very kind,' I smile, 'but you still have to go.'

He lunges – I try to duck, but he catches my head in his enormous hands and clutches my face lovingly towards his tender moist belly.

'I love you!' he cries, locking his fingers behind the back of my head and toppling backwards, vainly trying to use my head to regain his balance. My face is now approaching his crotch. He pulls my nose towards his piss-stained trousers. There is clearly no escape.

World War III

When the Third World War comes I'm going to be so sorted. No one is going to draft me off to be cannon fodder on some miserable mountainous front in the middle of nowhere, because I'll be tending you needy lot back home; and when western society crumbles under the military might of the developing world and their *Blue Peter* homemade chemical bombs, I shall have some of the most sought after skills on the post-holocaust market. For those of you who may require my services, I shall be somewhere in Kent and I would advise you to start stockpiling the tinned caviar and cigars now, because money won't mean a thing once the shops have all been blown up.

Seven of my patients in A&E have now claimed responsibility for the terrorist attacks in America, and I must confess I have taken a fairly free hand with my medical judgement and not called in the CIA. Generally, I think it's best to be straight with people, whatever they say, but it's also safer to be polite and non-confrontational if you want to avoid getting a knife in your thigh.

The latest, introducing himself as Elvis Presley, was very insistent.

'But you're the seventh person I've met this week who's said that,' I offer, hoping to broaden the conversation out as well as to gently challenge his opening gag. But he foils me straight off and lets the diagnosis out of the bag with his second line.

'Look,' he says, fingering his pockets and sneering. 'I'm mad and I've got a knife. OK?'

Now, it must be said that people who describe themselves as mad in A&E rarely are, much in the same way that people you meet at parties who describe themselves as bonkers are rarely not boring, particularly if they do unconvincing Elvis impressions every time you turn your back. Furthermore, people who really have knives usually just pull them out and have a go – or so I'm told by people much harder than me.

Having always been rather lucky with violent patients (and being generally a bit of a nice guy all round) I have to say that one of the greatest joys of A&E is seeing blokes the size of a shed come in with broken fingers from their latest thuggish exploit and having them be as charming as little pussycats. In fact, the only people who ever look like they might turn really nasty are the assertive middle-class self-advocates who expect you to work 'collaboratively' with them towards an 'optimum health outcome', as we say in the communication skills workshops.

Anyway, the main problem with people who come in pretending to have mental health problems when they're clearly just after a bed for the night or an admission to a psychiatric ward for their own amusement or something to do when nobody else is around to be interested in their personality disorder, is that it's really embarrassing when they turn out to be terribly ill. Particularly, I'm sure, if they end up hurting someone, and particularly if they've been telling you all along that that's their plan.

This, in fact, is the main problem with being an A&E doctor generally. You never see anyone for more than the opening stages of the game, and your main problem is to work out if they're ill, lame or just pretending. Take, for example, every junkie in the

South of England who's been in to see me, with their uncon-vincing stories of renal colic, demanding huge doses of opiates. Or take the Incredible Burping Man: he had been burping incessantly for a week.

'I think he's just got no manners,' suggested his girlfriend and I was inclined to agree, but he certainly was burping an awful lot. For all I know he died two hours after I sent him off home to see his GP.

So, as I ponder whether or not to take my terrorist punter seriously and wake up the mental health Crisis Response Team (whose idea of responding to a crisis is to turn up four hours later in matching black polo-neck jumpers) my punter reminds me of his plans.

'If you don't admit me to hospital,' he says, smiling, 'I'm going to blow up the motherfucker of all parliaments!' He smiles again. 'And then I'm going to find out where you live, "Doctor" Foxton, and blow that up too.'

Now, the idea of seeing Bedside Manor going up in smoke is one I find strangely appealing, but there are other doctors who live in hospital accommodation too, and for all I know some of them might quite like the old place. I tell my punter which psy-chiatrist is on-call and pop off to rouse the ironically named Crisis Response Team, but when I return he's done a runner. The nurses giggle as I fill the car park with police cars for the third time this week, but Elvis has definitely left the building.

Decide When You're Drunk

Some of you just don't know when to stop. It's been a month since anyone wanted to snog me and the first patient in the in-tray this morning had a huge red eye with which she could no longer see.

'Jizz,' she said, accusingly, as if it could possibly be my fault. 'Spunk. And it hurts like shit!'

I can't even begin to imagine getting up the energy for a direct hit these days, but the guy in the cubicle next door was determined to remind me of nature's bounty.

'Gung daan,' he mumbles incomprehensibly, speaking as if he had no tongue. I raise my eyebrows as he shows me the sticky mess on the floor of his mouth. 'Going . . .' – he winces and pauses – '. . . down.'

His girlfriend blushes as I look at the sharp edges on his lower front teeth and the thin, ripped frenulum that had once connected his tongue to the floor of his mouth. It is clearly severed and hideously infected. His glands are up, and he looks like he might have a temperature.

He has, rather manfully, developed pelvic inflammatory disease in his mouth, and I find myself thinking of the sexually transmitted diseases consultant I had when I was a student. He was perpetually infuriated, in the twilight of his career, by the lifestyles of his work-shy patients.

'They're all unemployed and they're just shagging all day. Of course they get bloody knob-rash. I don't know why they're so surprised. They'd get calluses on their hands too, if they ever did a day's work.'

Frankly, I can't imagine anything better than a life on the dole collecting interesting sexual injuries, but, sadly, the time has come for me to think about my career, choose a speciality, and apply for a proper job. Since I do my best thinking when I'm pissed, I sign up for the drug dinner and plough merrily through the unending pile of swollen ankles in anticipation of a bloodbath.

Drug dinners should be a patient's worst nightmare. The story goes like this: pharmaceutical companies employ a small army of flirtatious blonds (of both genders) whose job it is to get impressionable young doctors into a state of heightened drunkenness and arousal over an inevitable curry, and then subject them to a mind-control programme not unlike the CIA's experiments with LSD in the fifties.

They are paid according to how much we use their particular drug and will merrily deploy half-truths to this end, smiling sheepishly when caught out. We, on the other hand, are employed by the state to cure patients [*laughter*] without wasting the hard-earned cash of taxpayers such as yourselves. But we also like the drug reps' beer.

It is a veritable orgy of manipulation and deceit, and if we were ever sober enough to remember a single word they said, I'm sure this whole farcical process would adversely affect patient outcome. Suffice to say, however ropey our performance may be the morning after, getting drunk is the only way to ensure their advertising spiel doesn't stick in our memories, and so it is to your ultimate benefit.

I try to focus on the gynaecologist sitting next to me and probe him for careers advice.

'Forget it,' he mumbles. 'You'll spend your whole life negotiating hysterectomies with women who just don't like menstruating, retrieving lost condoms from foul alien landscapes with a pair of salad tongs and having *Guardian* readers at dinner parties getting all uppity about how you're medicalizing childbirth, when in reality it'll take a mother with a near-death experience to get you out of bed because the on-calls are so medieval.' Which all seems quite reasonable. 'And they'll all hate you because you're a bloke.'

'Get some of those stick-on sideburns, a nice jumper, and become a GP,' suggests my boss, at which point the doors of the curry house burst open and there, silhouetted against the moonlight, is the Incredible Boozing Man. This is a small town.

Two hours ago I'd caught him on the floor of the kids' cubicle in A&E, next to a pile of alcohol wipes, which he was carefully peeling, sucking dry, then discarding into a yellow plastic dumper truck being studiously wheeled backwards and forwards by a giggling toddler. I've never experimented myself, but I reckon you've got to work pretty hard to get drunk on alcohol wipes.

Now, the things that boozers do best, in no particular order, are (1) vomit, (2) beat up their wives and then cry about it, and (3) fall over. The restaurant owner, hearing the distinctive sound of the Incredible Boozing Man marauding through his establishment and greeting us all by name, appeared from behind a hidden door to be met with the smiling drunken faces of the people who had, just three nights previously, dealt with the memorable fall-out of his own drunken episode of wife-beating. At which point the waiter (whose wrists I sewed shut last week after a nasty argument with his girlfriend) sees the writing on the wall and does a runner back into the kitchen. We make our excuses, leaving the Quaxipram representative with the people who need her most.

The Death of the Incredible Boozing Man

It is always the embarrassing ones who die.

'I've taken twenty-four paracetamol,' she mumbles and looks at the floor of the cubicle.

My arse, I think to myself as I skim through a fistful of casualty cards recording this girl's nineteen previous attendances in A&E. There is no single occasion when she has managed to have a trace of paracetamol in her bloodstream.

So this is Munchausen's syndrome, kind of: ridiculous time-wasters who come in with pretend tummy ache or unconvincingly paralysed limbs or pathetic overdoses, and bugger us all about for a few hours. The Munch Bunch, as we like to call them.

'Stop wasting my time,' I say with a smile. She looks up, shocked, priming herself for a torrent of abuse. Surely somebody should think about referring this girl to the shrinks. I pull out a tourniquet and do my duty.

Other people are not so lucky. My friend, Stass, is up for a coroner's in a week because someone she sent home died the next day. You know what she did wrong? She apologized. Now the family is baying for blood.

Hospital managers, we are told, get rather upset with doctors who go around apologizing to patients over cock-ups. We tend to do it on the grounds that it makes everyone feel better and so it's just a nice way to end things. Unfortunately there are a few of you out there who can't cope with the uncertainties of life and our failure to have magical powers, and decide to try and make a few quid out of it.

Stass didn't stand a chance.

'She's just not quite right,' they said when they brought in the patient.

This is a common problem with elderly relatives, and your best bet is to find out when the family last saw them.

'Christmas,' they said. Nice way to treat your demented mother.

So you struggle on. 'In what way is she "not quite right"?' you ask.

They sneered, apparently, and pointed at her drooling. This is not such an unusual thing for an elderly woman to do when she has been abandoned by her family for ten months.

'Well, what was she like at Christmas?' asked Stass.

'Not drooling.'

What can you do? She looked like she might have had a bit of a urine infection. The medics didn't want to admit her, the family said they'd take her home and look after her, so off she went with some antibiotics . . . and died the next day.

Moments like this make you realize you're a grown-up. Fortunately, the Incredible Boozing Man doesn't have any family – apart from us – so there's nobody about to complain when we lose our patience and leave him at the bottom of the in-tray.

The last time he came in, I used him to teach the medical students about wound-healing: he comes in about three times a week after falling over drunk, so his head is a living demonstration model of the four stages of wound-healing, and it's all nicely slowed down by the booze. He will do anything to get booze.

I watch him sway into a cubicle, looking worse than ever, and pop down the corridor to grab a pair of gloves before examining his bloody head for the second time this week. As I walk back into the cubicle I catch him stuffing a bottle of Hibiscrub behind the trolley. He looks up at me guiltily.

'There is no booze in Hibiscrub,' I tell him, authoritatively. It's an old problem. Once we even got a call from the stroke rehab ward: 'There's some bloke up here drinking the Hibiscrub. Is he anything to do with you?'

'Yup,' we said. 'Send him down.'

So I feel my way around the Incredible Boozing Man's scabby head, trying to see through the grit and congealed blood for the freshest injury. There are a few to choose from, but in one place there's a step down and a step up. The bastard's got a depressed skull fracture – on my shift.

An hour later he was in the scanner. After one pass they saw the massive bleed and six hours later he was dead. Three hours after that we were in the pub, mourning our mascot, drinking like he would have – with a bottle of Hibiscrub on the table.

What a Hero

And then some junkie scumbag manages to pull his trousers down and take an overdose, right in front of me on the tube, at 10.30 on a Friday night. I mean, he actually unzipped his flies and spread his legs, right opposite me in the end carriage of a Central Line train, reached for his needle, pulled his filthy pants to one side and started rooting around in his groin for a vein. I only looked up from my book because of the stink. I was just up in town to see friends for Christ's sake.

Of course, like any other British person I averted my eyes and carried on reading. Needles don't bother me and neither do junkies, especially since I qualified and became the hardest man in the world. I just filed away a mental note that young people these days were shooting up in public on the tube instead of going to church.

Anyway, I happened to look up from my book just in time for that magical *Trainspotting* moment when he plunged in the needle and made a face like he was getting the world's biggest cuddle from a bounteous matriarch with a special thing for scabby smackheads; and then he threw himself into the air, jumped around for a few seconds, doing some pretty convincing fitting, fell to the floor, landed right on top of my feet and started frothing at the mouth and looking like he had definite plans to stop breathing.

The entire carriage freaked out. I remained seated, but shuffled my feet to the side of him. A girl to my left pulled the emergency alarm and shouted: 'Is anyone here medically trained?'

Now that's a very good line, I thought, and made a mental note to use it myself next time. Everyone was looking in our direction. I put my hand up sheepishly.

'OK,' she said.

It was at this point that it began to dawn on me that my dubious authority might well be undermined by my rather louche, retro, seventies party gear. It had never occurred to me that a pair of purple flared loon pants, a tight flowery polyester shirt and a big-arse paisley kipper tie that used to belong to my dad might impact negatively on my bedside manner. Surely all doctors looked like this thirty years ago?

But what was really undermining my confidence was not having an entire A&E department to hand, because, frankly, I'm pretty useless without one.

A crowd formed around us. 'What shall we do?'

'Nothing,' I said, smiling helpfully. They didn't look impressed. 'Well, I mean, he's just taken a bit too much heroin, and the only problem is if he stops breathing. In which case . . .'

– everyone watched him breathe attentively; there was no naloxone, no oxygen, no tubes and no anaesthetist – 'in which case, he's buggered,' I finished, and thought about kicking him to keep his attention focused on breathing, if the worst came to the worst.

'Why was he fitting?' piped up some clever Dick at the back of the class.

'No idea,' I said, smiling again. 'Interesting, isn't it?'

It's the kind of comment that would be quite normal in A&E. Everyone looked at me in horror. I was the only person in the whole carriage who wasn't standing around me, apart from the frothing junkie, who was lying on the floor, breathing.

And then, the million-dollar question: 'Can't we give him mouth to mouth?'

Well, I thought, looking down at the froth, I can answer that one quite easily. He was covered in spatters of blood. I lifted him gingerly into the recovery position with my feet. God knows where the needle was.

Finally, we get to the next station. People were shouting for an ambulance.

And then she arrives: the First-Aider. Panting.

'OK everybody,' she says. 'I'm a first-aider.' And dives on top of the patient. 'How long has he been here?' she barks. This, truly, is her moment of glory. She celebrates by sticking her hand right down inside his mouth, and has a good root around in there.

'I wouldn't touch him without gloves if I were you,' I say. 'He's covered in blood. And he might have AIDS.'

Everyone glares. I shut up. And the First-Aider starts ordering people around, with no apparent purpose, and refusing, infuriatingly, to let any of the London Underground staff move him, so we all have to stand around being late.

I sigh. The trouble with first-aiders is, they wait their whole lives for this special moment; and I hate to be a spoilsport, but they're slightly melodramatic. I blame it on the telly.

'If you put your hand in there once more,' I mumble, 'I swear he'll bite it off.'

Royal College Guidelines say don't stick your hand in their mouth without equipment unless you can see exactly what you're going for. But no one's listening. He's coming round, but she's not letting anyone move him until the ambulance arrives. I've waited for them before; I head for the sky and get into a taxi.

Suicide is Painless

My friend has killed himself. I mean, he wasn't really my friend. He was just some doctor I used to know. I can't even remember if I really liked him. But he killed himself, because of his job, because he was a doctor and because he felt awful and alone.

And because I know – from those times when I've been up all night, when I can hardly speak or walk properly from fatigue, and some relative is being rude to me, and I'm on the verge of tears, and some nurse is acting like I'm lazy because I went to see a patient on some other ward first instead of theirs, and I've got no senior support, and my boss is on my case, and I can see my whole career disappearing before my eyes unless I pull something superhuman out of the bag, and nobody understands – because I've been there, I know exactly, *exactly* how he felt. I feel right now that I know him all too well.

Doctors are really quite butch. I'm only telling you that in case you hadn't already worked it out. We're butch because, a lot of the time, everything in our lives is hellish, and we deal with it: if it's someone else's hell, we try to sort it out; if it's our hell, we just deal with it.

Maybe it's partly because we assume our problems can't possibly be as big as our patients', and maybe it's partly because we think problems are things that other people have and that we solve, and maybe it's also because there's just a spirit of 'chin up, stiff upper lip, firm resolve, and don't make a fuss'. Maybe it's because there's fuck all support. And then, maybe, it's just because there's simply no time in the days and the nights to make a fuss.

For example, this is how I found out that this guy was dead:

'Did you hear?'

'No.'

'Tim Forth's dead.'

'Really?' I raise my eyebrows, like it's clinical data.

'Killed himself.'

'Really?' I nod my head, sagely. We are with two girls. They are non-medics (that's a technical term).

So we hold forth, as amusingly as we can, about the daily hell of our jobs, the ridiculous abuse we get and the crazy working hours, and laugh about it as we compete for the most nightmarish on-call anecdote.

The girls don't believe the bit about the working hours, because no one ever does, so we have to explain, and do so with undisguised relish and pride, as their eyes widen. No, we're not making it up. And don't ever expect me to explain it to you again, because I'm bored of it.

'And I heard about someone else who killed themselves recently.'

I nod, as if only we could understand the pain, but it didn't really touch us.

'Apparently, a few days before it happened, he lost it one night in A&E, just went out into the waiting room and said, "Right, who here is in pain?" And only about half the waiting room put their hands up. And then he said, "OK, hands up: who's taken a painkiller?"' I smile at the prospect. 'And then, when only half of them kept their hands up, he announced, "Right, those of you who haven't taken painkillers can go home right away. And for everyone else, I'm sorry about the wait, but we're doing our bloody best!"' Cool. 'And he glared. Menacingly.'

I nod sagely. How can this man be dead? He was blessed with a vital insight into the lameness of the human condition and a strength of will far beyond the call of a poxy career in medicine. But he is – utterly dead: some bloke my age who felt awful and alone like I do half the time, but happened to have no mates that day. Was it pushy parents, barbaric working conditions or accidents of brain chemistry? Your guess is not as good as mine.

So if you're a doctor and you think it's all over and your whole world has gone irretrievably pear-shaped, I say this: Bail out. Don't kill yourself. Leave your job. Blow it out. Go on the dole. Do a few locums. Teach English abroad. Get a job in the city. Get a good night's sleep. Skive off sick. Reclaim your life: have it over again. You're young. You'll make new friends.

Anyway, I'm off to have a nice hot bath with the toaster. And even if I was never really friends with either of these two dead doctors: here's to you both, you poor, poor bastards.

The Trouble with Alternative Therapy

I hate all alternative therapists – largely because they're under-educated, malignant, jealous, greedy and manipulative liars.

That's what everybody likes to assume I think. Here I am, just a nice guy in a boring tie, trying to do the best for my patients and their terrible medical problems, by whatever means are most likely to work, who just happens not to find crystals or herbs very interesting, and you all think I'm a blinkered phallocrat on a science power trip, imposing his authority and maintaining the hegemony at the expense of his patients' holistic well-being. God, I hate alternative therapists.

So, I met this alternative therapist at a party and immediately she put me on the defensive. This happens a lot when you're a doctor at a party trying to get drunk – on one of the rare occasions when you're not actually working – and everyone else thinks you're attending as the earthly representative of an ancient and mysterious brotherhood which is, by turns, selflessly benevolent and intensely sinister. Generally, I can see it coming a long way off.

'So,' they say. 'You're a doctor?' The laser sights settle in on your forehead. 'Doctors told my mum she had the flu and she was dead from cancer in three weeks.'

My fault.

So this time, as the earthly representative of my people, I've managed to get an alternative therapist on my case, and she's spoiling for a fight. I cast around in my head for a conciliatory opening line that will present me as a broad-minded, intelligent, attractive and only slightly drunk junior doctor who is very interested in – but not unappealingly desperate about – snogging glamorous and feisty alternative therapists at parties.

'I just want whatever's best for my clients.' (Check that: I just said the word 'clients'.) 'I only really worry if I think they might be financially exploited,' I smile, winningly. 'Or emotionally manipulated,' I add, unconsciously, on autopilot. And then grit my teeth. The fact is, I've seen some patients get seriously done over by alternative therapists, although I could probably convince myself it was the work of a scurrilous minority in an unregulated industry. Obviously, the worst that usually happens is that someone hands over large sums of cash for a pile of fluff.

'Emotionally manipulated? What the fuck does that mean?'

She's fantastic, but I think I'm going home alone.

The problem, of course, is mutual jealousy. I am jealous of alternative therapists because they're privately employed by people with money to spare, which is obviously pretty yuck, except it means they can afford to spend absolutely ages talking to the patient and find out exactly where they're at and what they want. Bliss.

They, conversely, are jealous of us because most people take us seriously, and because they seem to think, like everyone else, that we all drive Rolls-Royces between our gentlemen's club and the on-call bedroom (with its manky NHS blankets and polyester sheets that spark in the dark). Oh, and because we don't believe a word they say.

But most of all, alternative therapists freak me out because half the time they do all the things they claim to hate most about doctors. Like getting all didactic and saying they know exactly what's wrong with someone and exactly what will make them better – when they clearly don't. Homeopathy for headache relief? That's not very holistic. Sounds to me like you're treating a symptom.

I revel in telling people that I don't know exactly what's wrong with them or whether or not a treatment will work, because I think it's good that people come to terms with the basic realities of science and probability and the fact that medicine is an inexact science where we tinker with relative risks. Particularly when they claim they want to get involved in the decision-making process or to have things explained as they really are.

There are exceptions to this. Sometimes patients will as good as say they want you to lie to them, and be certain and definite, and sometimes that's a fair enough part of the therapeutic relationship. Because, the thing is, mainstream medicine is often only really any good for the big problems like broken legs and heart attacks and cancer. For most of the small stuff, the stuff that is maybe mood congruent or has a major psychological component, we'd be lying if we said we could cure it. But they're still miserable, and maybe gently massaging in a placebo never did any harm.

That's what I really think. Is that so bad?

Well, I'm still single.

Just Another Night in Casualty

Dead babies. There are times when I despair. So I was just about to see this lady who had walked in with a sprained ankle and who had clearly mislaid her copy of the *Reader's Digest Guide to Commonsense Obviousness about Your Health*, because she hadn't taken any painkillers, when in came a blue baby in the arms of a screaming mother.

I like to imagine that nothing much can choke me up these days. Babies in general don't really do it for me. Terrified, screaming, desolate mothers, of course, are a whole different, gut-wrenching story.

When I cry [*places hand nobly on chest*], I cry for the human condition. And here it comes.

'You said I was next,' says Sprained Ankle.

'Excuse me,' I say, trying not to sweep her out of the way too obviously.

'No,' she says, and moves to block me. I try not to look too shocked and duck to the right.

'You said I was next!' she shouts. 'I've been here for eight hours!' I stare. 'Eight hours!'

An entire A&E department is converging on the resuscitation room. A man on oxygen and a large bleeping box is being wheeled out in a hurry. Someone has done a swift prioritization on the dead baby. Someone else hasn't.

'Eight hours!'

I feint to the left, then duck to the right; she blocks and catches me in the corner of the doorframe by the nursing station. I look inside for help, but all I can see is an agency nurse with minimal English who has clearly just called the wrong number for the paediatric crash team. It's only fifteen seconds since the blue baby arrived in casualty, but Sprained Ankle is more than a pain in the arse. I gently lever her against the wall and move in to call 222.

'Paediatric crash team to casualty, please,' I say, in my most urgent doctor voice. I listen to Tom put out the crash call over the bleep system in his favourite urgent-hospital-switchboard-operator's voice.

'Thanks Tom.'

'That's all right, Mick, pleasure mate,' he says. 'Anything else I can do you for? Free call to your sister in Australia?'

'Thanks,' I say, 'but I'm in the middle of a paediatric crash call.'

'So you are. Best of British.'

Sprained Ankle glares at me.

'You'll have to go back to the waiting room,' I say. And that is why it takes so long to get to see us in casualty. That and people who call ambulances for funny tingly feelings in their hands when they've got a hangover. That and years of underfunding.

'I'll see you as fast as I can,' I have often wanted to say. 'In the meantime, could you please fill out this form detailing every voting decision you've made over the past thirty years to show exactly how much you deserve it?'

My consultant, like all consultants in A&E, is the hardest man in the world. Once, he took a man who had been bullying the receptionist about waiting for several hours in to the resuscitation room and showed him five beds full of five exceedingly ill patients, and demanded to know: 'Which of these five people would you like me to boot out so we can urgently deal with the lump on your wrist?'

After the baby is pronounced dead (and God it is so screamingly awful) I go and smoke a cigarette outside on my own, and miss the consultant's touchy-feely pep talk. He catches me on the way out, and passes me a fraternal look.

I whinge about Sprained Ankle: 'Why can't people just get over the idea that we have some kind of open-ended commitment to their flakiest conditions?'

'We can't get rid of the open-ended commitment,' he says, 'as long as we want to sit on the moral high ground.'

I go back inside and get on with my night. There are no more dead babies.

At 5.30 a.m., astonishingly, unprecedentedly, it all goes quiet, and I lie down on a trolley for half an hour, to be woken up by a woman who has had a sprained ankle since the previous afternoon.

'I came now because I knew it would be much quieter,' she says.

Thanks a bundle, I think. And smile benevolently.

New Year's Eve

My registrar is not impressed that I'm thinking about becoming a psychiatrist.

'They're a bunch of boring, pretentious weirdos with no life who never answer their bleeps,' he says.

As he speaks, the cardiac arrest call goes out and we dash off to cubicle six. Actually that's not true. The cardiac arrest bleep goes off and I and the nurses dash off to cubicle six, while the registrar gives me his special it's-good-experience-for-you-to-run-arrests look.

The medical emergency we are faced with is as follows. The ninety-year-old man on home oxygen (who's had three strokes and two previous heart attacks) we needn't worry about for the moment, I can promise you: because half-dead ninety-year-old people with no quality of life who've decided to die can make the final push perfectly well on their own without any more broken ribs from the cardiac arrest team; because my hands will do the thinking in a resus quite happily without a brain until I have a heart trace to look at; and because the Good Lord, we can safely assume, has finally spotted all the dignified death opportunities He heartlessly neglected before this guy became bedridden, mute, brain dead and stuck in an oxygen mask all day. And you can't argue with the big guy.

No. The real medical emergency in this room, apart from my crushing indifference to death (I promise you that I'm perfectly competent and a very nice guy, but this old man's never coming back and it's going to be cruel trying), is the surgical house officer.

'I was just trying to do some blood gases,' she weeps. (She is properly crying.) 'And he went blue.'

Well, he's grey now, I think to myself. So get on with the chest

87

compressions. Who's the house officer around here anyway?

But she can't move. Which is a shame, because she's right in front of the heart monitor.

'Can you stand to one side, please? I can't see the monitor.'

That's not me speaking, by the way, that's the Advanced Life Support course instructor that lives in my head. My real brain doesn't start working until I see the trace, and it's a shockable trace: 'Stand clear.'

I look at the punter. He looks like a nice guy, even through the stroke. You can always tell by the time they're ninety. It would be nice, consequently, if we could avoid breaking any ribs until the medical registrar gets here to tell us to stop on grounds of futility.

I shock. The house officer winces.

This is very poor. Three shocks, no response, big surprise. In case I haven't mentioned it eight million times already, they never come back unless they're young, fit and healthy – so don't believe anything you see on *ER*.

'Carry on CPR,' says the ALS course instructor in my head, using my mouth. I look at the house officer pointedly. The best way to terminate a house officer freak-out, from my experience of having them, is to get on with it. She is frozen, apart from the sobbing.

Now check how holistic I am. My plan was that the teeny house officer did the chest compressions, and then we wouldn't have to break any ribs before the medical registrar got here to tell us to stop this charade. Unfortunately, the fear-ridden statue that now quakes before me means that the new, super-keen A&E nurse is going to do the chest compressions. He's built like a brick shithouse and ribs are cracking audibly. My master plan is foiled.

And so for the finale: the medical registrar arrived, then we stopped; then the patient was properly dead and then the pips went for midnight and it was 2002. So there we go.

The house officer – who now goes to bed at midnight (not in

my day, etc.) – buggered off and I smoked a fag and then saw seven billion drunks with eight zillion sprained ankles, had a poo, and went to bed in daylight.

Goodnight.

Advice for the Prince

Dear Harry,

Your dad has asked me to have a word with you about this drugs business, and seeing as how you're a prince and everything, I suppose I can let you in on a few secrets. By now you've probably worked out that you're not the only teenager in the world ever to drink beer and smoke a few jazz cigarettes.

And you obviously thought the people in that drugs clinic you politely smiled your way through were a million miles away from you and your friends.

Maybe.

Dope won't make your balls shrink, it won't make you grow breasts, it won't make you mad, it won't make you stupid and it won't make you into a raging heroin addict. It might make you a bit of a lazy teenager if you do it every day, which you already know, but you probably think that the worst thing about cannabis is that you can get busted for it.

You're almost right. A hundred thousand peaceful dope smokers get busted every year under the Misuse of Drugs Act, and have their career plans ruined by a criminal record. Lots of them end up moaning in GP clinics about their crap lives, but in your line of work, whatever that's supposed to be, I suppose that might not be a problem.

The thing is, Harry, you've got to learn to spot the difference between drug use and drug abuse early in life these days. Not everyone who drinks is an alcoholic. Dope doesn't lead to heroin any more than alcohol leads to darts, and anyone who tells you otherwise just doesn't understand statistics: surveys might show that people who smoke cigarettes have more sex, but when I want a shag I don't go out and cane my way through forty Rothmans with an optimistic glint in my eyes.

Here's the point: I can still remember the day my best friend came home and said, 'I've had a shit day: I need a spliff.' At the time, I'd almost have preferred it if he'd charged into the kitchen and shouted 'Hey, I've got a big bag of crack, everyone, and I plan to have some fun!' I don't know if I stand by that, after what I've seen, but I know that was the first time I ever worried about drugs.

Because using drugs to cope is a really bad trip to get on, and it creeps up on unhappy people. I can see now that how and why you use drugs is much more important than which ones you use, and you've been through the mill, Harry, old boy. I reckon maybe you're at risk.

Smoking dope might be a poor predictor of heroin use and alcoholism, but I'll tell you some good ones: loss of a parent; parental discord; disjointed home life; stress; no direction. And I'll tell you some more bad signs: taking drugs and drinking on bad feelings, self-medicating to try and make them go away; drinking or taking drugs secretively. And it's worse that you have to – because you don't get proper advice or sensible role models.

And here's a good one: getting properly out of your head and being unimaginatively abusive. There is no excuse for calling one of the pub workers a 'fucking frog'. Bad scene.

Don't get confused, Harry. You're an opinion former and a role model. Just because every right-thinking person these days thinks alcohol and cannabis should be available without prohibition handing the market over to gangsters and locking up nice innocent people, that doesn't mean they're necessarily harmless.

And likewise, just because drugs have their dangers, that doesn't mean we should let individual users and society blame all their problems on them. I've lost count of the number of drug abusers (and that's abusers, not users) who've said, 'Its the dealers, doc. I blame the pushers.' Bollocks. People have problems. And they can have them with alcohol, heroin, cannabis or tranquillizers from their GP.

I'm not going to tell you that drugs are bad, because you'll just look at me like I'm your dad in that clinic and ignore every word I say. But you've just got to watch yourself, Harry. Because everybody else is. It's best that you don't take drugs and alcohol, but if you really have to, at least do it sensibly, for everyone's sake. And if you ever need a chat, find a nice sensible doctor.

Four Days to Go and I'll Be a Psychiatrist

Sometimes it's the sheer stupidity of some people that astonishes me – mainly my own, in choosing a job that stops me ever seeing my friends in return for a boatload of abuse off the public every day and twenty-four grand a year. But also my registrar, for thinking he's the hardest man in the universe.

'Just get the laughing-gas mask back and boot him out. He's a scag-head.'

It's important for you to know that my extremely posh registrar only ever deploys street slang like this with an ironic smirk on his face, in order to reinforce his image as the hard man of emergency medicine. And it is, as ever, an astute assessment of the clinical situation.

Because the extremely smelly man in the next cubicle (who looks very much like a heroin addict pretending to have renal colic) is not the one-in-a-thousand genuine punter we always diligently check for, but, in fact, another heroin addict pretending to have renal colic: what is more, he couldn't even be bothered to learn the story properly. And the A&E sister recognized him as a repeat offender. And he has ID in his pocket for the name she remembered him by.

This man isn't just a crap actor. He has been actively mocking me, and he thinks he can get away with it, for the simple reason that he is twice my size. He also won't give the nitrous mask back, even when I use my special doctor's voice. The nurses are suddenly too busy to help.

'Fine. If you all want to be pussies about it, as usual, then I'll go in there and be nurse, security guard and registrar, shall I?' My registrar flounces off.

Sister curtsies. 'Lord Earl to see you, Dr Foxton.'

Lord Earl is an elderly homeless Rastafarian who smells of urine and comes in about once a week when people beat him up for fun – because you are fundamentally a pretty sick bunch out there. That is all anyone knows about him. Just ask the social workers about it if you're worried. This is A&E for fuck's sake.

'All right, Earl?' I say.

'Irie, doc.'

He is carrying a bunch of rags in front of him. 'Take a seat.'

He hasn't even been through triage, but everyone is nice to Earl. It's traditional. He just walks in and helps himself.

'Might have to lie down, doc.'

'Right you are, Earl,' I smile. He pulls away the rags.

'Got a bit of a problem this time, doc.'

He's a dead man. I think I can see bowel hanging out through the blood.

I press on the hole and shout for help and hear my registrar roar in reply. It turns out that he had managed to pull the nitrous-oxide mask off the junkie, but when he leaned over to turn off the tap, he felt a jaw dripping in HIV-laden saliva clamping down on his ear.

'I want that fucker arrested right now,' he whispers to sister as we call anyone we can think of to come and sort out Earl.

In four days I'll be a psychiatrist. Which I reckon I'll be pretty good at. So seven hours later, at 1 a.m., a seventeen-year-old French exchange student potters into A&E talking bollocks in an outrageous French accent.

'I feel so strrrrange. I can't explain it, everything feels just so unreal.' The triage nurse has already warned me that she's not going to shut up about it and go home. 'It's just all – so much more detail, and my heart is racing and I'm caught in my thoughts and other people and every possibility must be calculated for, every . . .' All right. This isn't an existential counselling service.

'Can you think of anything that might explain it?' I ask, patiently.

She starts to giggle. 'Well, it's another thing. I . . .' She giggles uncontrollably. She can't even open her eyes, let alone string words together.

'Where have you just come from?' I ask, bored senseless.

'. . . Party!' she squeals, and bends over crippled with laughter.

'Did you take any drugs there?'

I try to look like nobody I know has ever even thought about taking drugs, though chilled enough so that it's OK to tell me.

'No.' She laughs. 'Oh, my God!' She grabs my arm and nearly falls off the trolley. 'But I ran out of proper cigarettes and somebody gave me a roll-up one.' She takes of her pink sunglasses, which are blood red, and squeals with laughter.

'Are you feeling hungry?' I sigh.

She stops laughing and stares with immense gravity. '*Merde!* Do you have any popcorn?'

I can barely be bothered to write in the notes.

'You're stoned,' I smile. 'Just go home.'

Psychiatry

Paranoia

The last thing I remember, I was delivering babies and drinking beer all day at medical school. Suddenly I'm a psychiatrist. I'm even wearing a tweed jacket. I wander past some muddy Portakabins in yet another shitty NHS facility in the Home Counties and try to find outpatients with a photocopied map from the postgraduate centre.

So for those of you who don't know, psychiatrists are doctors. Which is partly because we prescribe drugs, and partly a reflection of a phallocratic and prescriptive medicalization of reality, sanity and normalcy that is a devious and undeserved historical relic. Or at least I suppose that is a thesis of yours that we may end up having to consider at length. Hey, check it out: I'm paranoid already.

Psychiatrists don't do psychotherapy like Frasier, or at least baby psychiatrists don't, and I can tell you this with absolute confidence because I am one and I don't know how to, and neither does anybody else I know. But I don't want to say too much and undermine the whole show. I mean, what if our power, or rather [*clears throat*] our therapeutic efficacy, is born of an illusory confidence? I'm fine. I'm a pretty nice guy. I loved psychiatry at medical school. I want so badly to be good at it.

This is the sound of me trying to convince myself it's going to be OK, smoking a fag outside outpatients before I go in to meet my predecessor for the handover. I drop a half-smoked cigarette into the mud. Mainly because I am shitting myself.

'Hi. Mike, I'm Conrad.'

Conrad is the most perfect thing I have ever seen. He is immaculate. He radiates confidence. He looks about thirty-two. He looks like he can do anything. I am a fraud.

'I've got a couple of people here I wanted you to meet before we change over,' he says. 'They're a bit fragile; they don't like change much. And I reckon one or two of them will probably cut in the next week, what with us changing over.'

Cut? Cut their arms? Make cuts in their arms and leak blood, because I'm starting? Jesus Christ. I smile understandingly. I have to get out of here.

'So, shall I show you around quickly and then introduce you to the patients?'

No. I don't want to meet the patients. I'm terrified of the patients.

'Great.' I smile weakly. 'Thanks.'

So once again I meet seventeen secretaries whose names I will never remember and once again he tries to get me to meet the patients.

'Sure,' I say, smiling. I am a fraud. 'Just run me through out-patients quickly. What . . . ground do you usually cover?'

He looks up. 'Oh, shit,' he says. 'It's your first job.'

Yes. And I am a fraud. So he tells me about outpatients and I write it all down, and I remember I don't even remember how to do a mental state examination properly or any side effects of any drugs or how to do a risk assessment or how sections work or what schizophrenia really is. Because I am a fraud.

'It's fine,' he says. 'Psychiatry: six diagnoses, twenty drugs. It's fine.' He smiles perfectly, with perfect teeth. 'There are no psychiatric emergencies. Take your time. Find your feet. Ask for help. Just be nice. Smile a lot. Don't run over time. Just do what you do. All psychiatrists are weirdos anyway. It's fine.'

Conrad is not a weirdo. He is perfect. I want him to stay with me for ever.

But you see, it's a funny thing about being a doctor: people plonk you down in appalling situations with minimal training and wait for you to come up with the goods. Medical school, which is frankly a farce, was at best a subliminal education where at some stage, from these vast oceans of factual sludge, you manage to extract a representative and intuitive background idea of how things should work in the body. Then you supplement this with the practical stuff about what you really need to know to be a doctor, usually at 3 a.m. when you're the only person around with even half a clue and all the punters kick off at once and the registrar is in bed. The system works. It works fine. Just don't worry about it. I don't any more.

'The boss is away at a conference for a week,' says Conrad. 'In fact he's usually away. That's a good thing, it means you have a lot of autonomy and you learn faster. Here's your bleep.' I am now under remote control. 'And here's your attack alarm.' He presses a button and fills my ears with pain for half a second. 'Pull this pin when the crackheads kick off and five academic secretaries in their fifties will come rushing to your rescue. Let's go and meet the punters.'

It's Normal to be Scared

'Where's your panic button then?'

He's about ten feet tall, but kind enough to lean over and put his huge ugly mouth right in front of my nose.

'I'm sorry?' I smile, while he stares intently at me with funny red eyes. To be fair, there's something a bit put-on about this aggression, but I start shitting myself just to be on the safe side and take a casual look around the room. Nobody's told me about any panic buttons. I probably should have asked before I started clinic. 'I don't think there is one,' I say casually, my relaxed manner implying that nothing could be less needed at this moment, what with how unthinkable it would be for any patient to try to attack a nice, cuddly, chilled-out, first-week-on-the-job psychiatrist like me.

'Don't fuck about, I know you've got them. And where's your personal attack alarm?' He bends his enormous frame around to scan my belt from all angles while asking this second, extremely good, question.

'I think I left it on the kitchen table. I don't like them,' I say, as he starts doing something funny with his eyes to imply that he's so mad he thinks he could get away with killing me in return for a few relatively tolerable years in a nice forensic secure unit. 'I don't think I need one.' I smile hugely. I am so chilled. I repeat it to myself. I am so chilled . . .

He wrinkles his nose and stares incredulously at me. Maybe he's thinking I'm too stupid to be worth crippling.

'I'm a nice guy,' I shrug. 'I smile a lot. No one wants to hit me.' I smile some more. This is a mind-control trick I learned watching *Star Wars*. He shrugs and sits down.

'Can I smoke?' he asks. Clearly the answer is no. I open the window.

'Of course,' I smile.

Not bad, I think: it's my first clinic, and I may be failing to maintain barriers, but I still have my looks and the use of my legs.

But I don't have a lighter: and so my potential mass murderer, who only sat down five seconds ago, sighs and gets up to go and find one.

'Wait . . .' I say, trying to think of a way to re-engage him, so I can work out if it's just me he wants to scare or if I have a protective duty to society that needs discharging.

'Wait . . .?' He gazes out of the window and turns his head to stare back at me wearily, like he can barely stomach my ham-fisted attempts to negotiate a good rapport. 'Good one,' he snorts, quietly contemptuous, and shuts the door behind him.

I pick up my pen professionally and prepare to frame the events of the preceding two minutes in the notes: *SHO outpatients, 23/2/02. Patient seen alone. Threatened to attack me and left immediately. Disappointed with self. Don't know what to do. No one to ask. What am I doing here? Shit. Foxton.*

And then the gravity of the situation starts to trickle in. My consultant's away, I'm the only psychiatrist in a clinic in some middle-of-nowhere provincial town and a patient has just come in, threatened to attack me, then walked out on to the streets.

I feel dizzy under the evil fluorescent lights. He has gone now, and there's no way I can get him back. He's out there some-where. I stare at the wall in front of me. It's getting closer. I swear they all are.

Why didn't I section him? I wouldn't even know how to. I'm so alone I feel short of breath. I stare at the blank page in front of me. I couldn't even get him to answer my questions. I didn't even ask them.

What if he kills someone? I didn't even ask him if he was going to. I want to puke. He's probably doing it right now. He's probably got a knife in his pocket. He's probably sticking it in some little old lady. Oh shit. It'll be on the telly. Should I call the police? Oh shit. And they'll say I saw him on the day he did it and I did nothing. Oh shit.

I Just Need a House with Electricity

The biggest problem my punters have got is you lot.

'My kids don't want to know me. This place is all I've got.'

This place is a miserable suburban day centre for people with chronic mental health problems where I see one person a week. At least I think it is. It's so smoky I can hardly see my own glasses.

'Philip?'

When Philip smokes, the cigarette never moves more than a fingerprint away from his lips. It doesn't seem to involve any movement in the upper limb. I've been watching them all closely over the past few weeks and I think it's the cigarettes that move by themselves.

Philip is a financier's dream: he can turn a new washing machine and a few pairs of trousers into a £15,000 debt in five years flat. If you're looking for new markets, these are the boys you should be targeting. He's suggestible and desperately aspi-rant, but more than that, he still has a trail of smoke wisping out of his yellow moustache. Either that or his face is on fire. I decide to give it a minute and see what happens.

'I'm so embarrassed.'

He is, and it's painful. One of you out there has made this man feel very stupid. 'It's just really depressing. I only wanted to be . . . normal, you know. It's pathetic, isn't it?' He's so resigned and natural with this insight that it almost feels like the most natural response would be to nod and agree. 'I didn't even need the washing machine. It was huge. Anyway, it's broken now. I have to go to the launderette, which I don't like because it makes me paranoid. I don't like people looking at my clothes.'

I'm looking at his clothes. He would be pretty cool if he were seventeen. And maybe black.

'Nothing looks normal on me.' Enormous denim skater pants and 'phat' white trainers certainly don't. He's forty. 'I bought these trousers last week when I went out shopping with the carer who comes to the house. She told me they looked good. Why can't people just be straight with me? God, I get so depressed.'

I prepare to pounce. Depressed: suicide. The most definitive negative outcome in any psychiatric patient. Suicide risk is the one thing I have been told to document every time I see someone, even if I manage nothing else.

'How low do you get, at your lowest?' I throw out as an opener.

'You lot are obsessed.' He looks at the ceiling. 'I'm not going to kill myself, all right? I suppose that means I don't get a community nurse.'

Jesus. These guys know more about the psychiatric system than I do.

'Of course not.' I smile. But you're not answering my question, I think, and I need to write down the answer. Because for some reason, somebody, possibly a lawyer, has decreed that me writing it down now will make a difference if you decide to kill yourself later.

'Well, I'm not going to say it. Anyway, they've cut off my electricity, so I can't electrocute myself.'

Small mercies. I don't think he's going to kill himself. I call the social workers. Well, that's not quite true. Prepare yourself for exactly how boring my job is: I call the social workers on the number Philip has been trying, but all I get is some kind of voicemail. I call the number on the voicemail and get some kind of fax machine.

'Yup. That's right. That's the one.' He looks out of the window. I call the other number for the social work team and get Vivaldi. 'And the kids on the estate keep throwing things at me. They spat on my trousers this morning.'

I smile understandingly. We both look at the large greasy mucous stain on the front of his trousers. This man needs a new wardrobe and a house with electricity on an estate full of *Guardian* readers.

Finally we get through to Marjorie. I try not to be shitty about the fact that it took twenty minutes.

'Oh yeah. Artramont Estate, I suppose?' she asks.

I look up. 'Artramont Estate?' Philip nods.

'Jesus,' she says. 'There's some kid working for one of those new electricity companies who went round door-to-door signing up all the clients whose finances we have to manage. Now we don't know where any of the bills are going. He's a pushy little fucker by the sound of it.' Sounds about right. 'Has he got anywhere else to go? We might have to take him into hospital.'

Surely this isn't cost effective. Surely this isn't psychiatry. I look up wearily and catch myself dead. Philip is crying.

Suicide is Painful

So at 3 a.m., because it's always 3 a.m., and because somehow the clientele know that it wouldn't really work so well presenting Suicidal-on-the-Bus to casualty at three in the afternoon on a sunny day, I am called from the sparking acrylic sheets of the on-call room by some grumpy A&E doctor.

'This is it. I've had enough. I'm going to kill myself. I've planned it all out. You've got to admit me.'

It's one of the peculiarities of modern life and the far-sightedness of the human psyche that this is the patient speaking, rather than the overworked overstressed and underpaid SHO in A&E.

Suicide rates fall in wartime.

Right. Now there are a few things you should know about how hard-hearted I'm about to be. First, everyone is suicidal these days and not all of them can come into my hospital because there's no room at the inn. This is a decision you all made collectively in the 1980s when I was about twelve years old so it's no good moaning to me about it now. Second, feelings are my business these days, and however cuddly I might appear on the outside, I'm paddling away frantically like a scheming little duck underneath the tranquil waters of my heart-warming smile. Just dig it.

Suicide is the big concrete negative outcome in psychiatry, not to mention a king-size tragedy. It's up there with murder and it makes us all shit our pants or at least it does me because I'm only a baby psychiatrist. So let's tighten our sphincters, loosen our ties, polish our smiles and knock up a quick crystal ball to predict whether or not she really is going to kill herself if we boot her out on to the streets just because you lot voted in Thatcher for twenty years.

Risk assessment is all in the demographics, the previous, and the mental state. Young women with friends, in general, don't kill themselves; they just pretend. Grumpy old bachelors, they really go for it. The closest they get to seeing a psychiatrist is when they're sloshing around in a big dish on a slab in the mortuary underneath the on-call bedrooms. Which makes a bit of a mockery of my job. Think how we feel about it.

I ask how she has been feeling recently.

'Awful. I'm crying all day and I can't sleep. I'm tired all day,

I've lost my appetite and I can't concentrate on anything. Oh, and its always worse in the morning.'

Amazing. So matter-of-fact. And a full set of biological symptoms of depression in the first paragraph. I focus on being relaxed and understanding. Even if it's a put-up job, she has still got to be pretty unhappy, and it's not her fault I've got to work all day tomorrow. Every contact should be therapeutic. Grit your teeth.

'How's your self-esteem?'

'Low. I just feel so helpless and hopeless. And worthless.' This girl knows Beck's triad of depressive cognitions better than I do. 'And guilty.' Bingo. Full house. 'And I live alone.' She can read my mind. Or she reads psychiatry textbooks. No one to keep an eye on her. Very bad sign. She so knows it. The gun is in my chest. My hands are above my head. The only question is: what's the ransom? A fistful of benzos? A week on the inside?

I look up her previous on the computer and she has fifty-six presentations to this A&E alone, all either teeny overdoses or threats. It's a blatant personality disorder, a world of frustration, untreatable, incessant, lifelong maladaptive, manipulative anxiety-inducing nightmare punters from hell. I just don't get them. I think that's because nobody does. I think you're sup-posed to have firm boundaries. I think that means not admitting them. I think that means having balls ten times the size of mine.

I call the registrar.

'Sweet thing,' she says. 'First night on-call? Much love.'

When did an orthopaedic registrar ever talk to me like this? I present my tiny balls.

'Oh, honey. This will grumble on for years. She might kill herself one day, but you have to send her home or ask yourself, what will you achieve with this admission?'

She's so sane. And the answer is, rather obviously, that I don't want someone to go home and kill themselves on my first night on-call. At any cost. I'm so lame.

'Oh, such a dearest thing,' she coos. 'Have a bed. For both of you. Goodnight. Oh, bless. Sweet thing. Goodnight.'

And I'm in love.

Just Hand Over the Drugs

'I want my grandma to have the pills that stop you being grumpy. I know you've got them, because you gave them to my sister, so you needn't fuck about.'

I smile placidly and plot out my conciliatory riposte before digging about for a bit more background. But the seeds of doubt are planted. Maybe that is all I do: just dish out the happy pills. They don't seem to make many of you very happy.

'That's because they don't address the root cause.' Suddenly a chorus of sanctimonious liberals appear stage left, dressed in pink and blue monopoly money and dancing under candy-coloured spotlights. 'They should all have individual therapy!' they chime in unison.

'That might be a bit expensive for a condition with a lifetime incidence of 10 per cent,' I suggest nerdishly, pensively plucking a few notes off one of their costumes. One of the more attractive cash fairies dances over and rubs my nose flirtatiously, but in a slightly patronizing fashion.

'Oh, you sweet silly thing . . . ' she squeals.

'Well?' And I am, in fact, in clinic, under striplights.

So I push the point as far as I dare with the scariest grand-daughter in the world, and of course our poor old grumpy grandmother is in fact as depressed as hell. Everyone she's ever known is either dead or the depressed and unemployed product of her ancient loins living on a hellish council estate, and she doesn't want anything apart from some tablets to take in the evenings because she markets herself to herself as a coper who wouldn't want to trouble a counsellor. Obviously it's my job to dish out the drugs and shut up, so I dish out the drugs and smile obediently.

I probably should have introduced them to the next patient.

'Your tablets gave me a tummy ache.' He glares at me, wounded and angry, like I'm the most evil bastard he's ever met in his life. Take note: if this were a husband–wife relationship, instead of a doctor–patient one, I would at this point turn around in a huff and say something like, 'Well, I was only doing my best to help. I shan't bother next time.'

I look back at the notes. My predecessor didn't even think the patient was depressed and throws the word 'dysthymia' about in the summary. Dysthymia means you've just always been a bit of an unhappy person. The only thing that drugs do, as far as I can tell, is get them out of the clinic room on time for the next patient to come in.

I try and ask him how he spends his days, partly to get a bit of friendly chat going and partly to find out if he does anything at all.

'These drugs are useless,' he says. 'I'm still clinically depressed.'

I ask about daytime energy.

'How long have you been a psychiatrist?'

Right. That's below the belt. I'm a perfectly nice guy, I know all the stuff in the books and all my lovely depressed patients this morning were very nice to me and I was very nice back to them and now suddenly you are being a bastard for no obvious reason. I start to sweat and mumble an explanation for my questions that ends up sounding like an apology, while he glares at me. What am I apologizing for?

Because it's my fault he's unhappy. Because I am a crap psychiatrist. I have no idea what to do.

I concoct a lame excuse to leave the room and call Conrad, my perfect predecessor, from the phone next to the loo. I explain the situation and struggle to make a joke out of it.

'Conrad. Help me. My patients are making me have feelings I don't understand.'

He laughs. 'Well, don't expect any support from the boss. Isn't he pretending to be at another academic conference this week?' The consultant didn't tell me he was pretending to be at an academic conference this week. I've only met him about three times. I think he might be deliberately avoiding me.

'Boundaries, Mike,' says Conrad. 'Just document the non-existent suicide risk, increase the dose and get him out of the door as fast as you can.'

'Is this counter-transference?' I ask, lamely.

'I don't care what they call it. You're doing fine. Regain the control you need without being controlling. Accept your feelings, but hide them and try to understand them later. And remember, just because he's a psychiatric patient, that doesn't mean he can't also be a prick.'

The Boys in Blue

Now that I've got a job in medicine where I don't have to wash my hands before I go to the toilet, it's easy to forget all that boring stuff about physical medicine. But patients who were banged up in the old-style psychiatric bins for their whole lives have ten years shaved off their life expectancy and, apart from the fact that they all smoke about eighty fags a day, nobody can tell you why.

I'll tell you why. It's because the drugs are all dirty and they've got junior psychiatrists like me, with all the postgraduate experience of a medical student, having to play at being GP for all their physical problems during weekends on-call, and usually during the week too.

So I have a quick flirty moan with the girl from Saturday night (she's so fine) as we hand over the bleep on a sunny Sunday morning, until I get called to go and look at two rashes on the ward.

'Do you think it could be erythema purpuginosa?' asks the nurse. 'That's why I called you.'

I don't remember much about erythema purpuginosa. In fact, I'm pretty sure it doesn't even exist, but smile anyway because in some hospitals when you're on ward cover and it's quiet, the single nurses will bleep you for trivia just to check out the junior doctor totty. And frankly, miles away from any big cities out here in the M4 corridor of London's party, I don't get many opportunities to meet girls my age.

Suddenly some bloke twice my size shoves a drug chart between my face and her breasts: 'Sign here.'

I see *Lorazepam 4mg* scribbled on the front. Sounds like an awful lot of benzos to me.

'She's kicking the shit out of Brendan and she's a drug-abusing personality disorder who never settles with less than 4mg.'

We both look out of the nursing station window at a scuffle which I have no desire or training to be a part of. Nurses deal with that, and I have no idea why or how they do it. In America, you know, they don't stand for it. People get tied up. It's not a reflection on whether patients are bad people, it's about normal people being able to do a proper job without getting assaulted. I'm glad it's not my decision, because it's an ugly one.

But first-line management of aggressive behaviour is containment and seclusion, I suggest.

'You're new, aren't you?'

I smile, because I can't think of anything else to do.

'There are only four nurses on this ward today. Two of them are agency.'

I think he's being helpful.

They jab the assailant in the bum and she starts smiling because that nice warm benzo feeling is a great way to reward really aggressive behaviour, while I flick through the notes. This nasty piece of work with a personality disorder has been kicking the shit out of the same vulnerable five-foot schizophrenic man twice a week for a month. If you're going to have that sort of thing going on then, frankly, there's no point in building your hospital in the first place. What's more, there is absolutely no reason why plenty of people with psychiatric diagnoses can't be held responsible for their actions.

I flick through her notes and find an explicit entry from some eminent consultant: *In conclusion, it would be both appropriate and therapeutic that this woman should be held legally responsible for her actions. Particularly assault.* My intuition is vindicated. I call the fuzz.

The boys in blue appear and manœuvre around the ward, being uninterested but polite to everyone and showing no intention whatsoever of pursuing any charges. I suspect it may have something to do with a woman hitting a man, until I hear the phrase 'pair of mentalists' and a bit of giggling.

Now I'm the first to say that professionals who work in difficult situations can be real human beings with real human responses and you can't keep up a godly front all day every day. I'm not surprised if policemen dislike drug-takers or burglars more than *Guardian* readers do, what with all the abuse and beatings they get off them. But *pas devant les enfants*, darlings. And please don't just saunter off and leave this woman stomping around with her unboundaried sense of invulnerability. I prescribe a therapeutic arrest.

Of course, the fuzz tell the nurse they probably won't be pursuing the matter 'but it's all on file', studiously avoid eye contact with me, and make for the door, when I feel a wave of self-righteousness gathering force inside me. I square up and put on my serious face.

'Look. She hit him and she's competent to face charges. Who's the psychiatrist and who's the policeman? You start assessing competence on the day I start spraying black people with CS gas.'

Well that's what I'd like you to think I said. But you can't fight that kind of battle alone on a Sunday afternoon with a moderate hangover when you're just a little baby SHO psychiatrist, so I traipse back to the on-call room and watch the *EastEnders* omnibus, on my own, with a cup of tea.

Victor the Drunk

OK, now I'm really paranoid. First, I am absolutely convinced that my last patient was recording our session together, because he kept asking me why I was asking certain questions, and then angling his lapel towards me. And he definitely had a wire trailing down the inside of his jacket. And he kept fiddling with a Walkman-shaped object in his pocket. And if that wasn't enough, you're all watching me and listening to my thoughts, and now the only other psychiatrist ever to write in about this column tells me I'm 'a fascinating case study in counter-transference'.

Counter-transference, for those of you who don't know, is the name psychiatrists invented for the funny feelings our patients make us have. As in 'I get amazing counter-transference from Mr Bartlett. He's so good at eliciting feelings of anger in the people he meets.' Or as in 'Maybe I should get out of this job before I develop some kind of really serious neurotic disorder diagnosed by someone writing in to the *Guardian*.' Apparently it's funny that working in an unsupported psychiatric job in the middle of nowhere with a frequently absent locum consultant is starting to do my head in.

So, everybody has their favourite patients: someone they review just that little bit too often or stick in among the difficult patients because they're interesting or good company. And this is true, all you clever old psychiatrists out there, whether you admit it to yourselves or not. Thank God I've booked in Victor this morning.

Victor, international man of mystery turned tragic boozer, has lost none of the faultless charm and witty repartee with which he once reigned supreme in several of Soho's most famous drinking dives, although he has lost a wife and children to some rather determined alcohol abuse along the way. He has also become a compulsive gambler, and now lives a rather grotty life here in the Home Counties, 'playing the ponies'.

Now, psychiatry is full of epic and tragic tales of human weakness, and a pissy market town is certainly a fitting backdrop for them, but I've been secretly hoping I could at the very least help Victor to have a bath and get sloshed in Knightsbridge again, instead of his crummy bed-sit. So inevitably I've been upping the dose of Quaxipram every week or so, in return for ten minutes of prime anecdotal material delivered in a faultless upper-class Peter Cook accent. But Victor is going seriously downhill: and all he will talk about is the money he's lost on the horses.

So, what is the job of a psychiatrist? I just dish out drugs and do risk assessments for admission to hospital, don't I? I mean, we have all these elaborate fantasies and make a point of being serious and emotionally flat with our patients, so that we can be a blank slate and have a relationship unlike normal social ones, so they have nothing to lose by telling us everything and we can both duck this 'transference' stuff. But I am clearly no analytic psychotherapist.

However (and bear with me here) I am quite definitely of the opinion that Victor – who endured an early life riddled with such unspeakable and unjust horrors that he has been quite understandably scarred ever since – with this gambling, this unending torrent of self-inflicted, crippling financial blows, with this self-imposed, homemade misery, this guy is collecting injustices.

Now, I'm not about to go out, buy a couch, grow a beard and start rambling on about ids and superegos, but the question is: do I share my limited insight with Victor? Or do I stay on home territory and up the Quaxipram?

In a flash of insight I decide to try and lead him gently into exploring the issue himself. I ask him what he's expecting to find when he goes to the tracks, his frame of mind when he leaves the house, what he expects will happen there.

'I don't go to the tracks any more,' he looks at the floor. 'I do it all on the Internet now. I only leave the house to buy drink. Or . . . pills.'

And so, it turns out, I've missed the boat in a big way: he's going to kill himself and has been planning it all week. No food. He's been double-locking the door and lining up the packs on the kitchen table and rolling the pills in his hands and thinking about whether he can hold out until this moment right now when he comes to tell me because I, apparently, can help. Which is more horrifying than it is touching. I ask the right questions, but he has got the classic demographic for a successful suicide; he's absolutely intending to do it, and there is no way to avoid an admission. Bugger analysis: how do I find a bed manager at half five?

On My Own and Out of My Depth

'I've been negotiating with the Tate. I'm going to curate a room.'

So clearly he's quite mad. And I can see the way you're looking: you think I'm about to play this man for laughs. My second-favourite patient.

You absolute scumbags. You underestimate me. The truth is so much more sinister.

I love patients with mania because they make me feel alive. It's depression's glitzy alter ego, way off the end of the happiness scale and into sheer beaming grandiose wonderfulness: born on Broadway, destined for the stars, the world at its feet, mania can take you anywhere, but usually into debt and depression. Like when you remortgage the house to buy that thirty-foot yacht you deserve, and then come down and realize what a big fat mess you've made.

Mania took Phil on a mission to London.

'Yeah, the Tate are pretty keen on me.' He crosses his legs professionally and puts his hands behind his head. 'And they want me to curate a room.' Sounds great. He's got the biggest smile on his face. 'No really. It's true. I've counted, right, and they've got six of those big monochrome paintings. Six! The ones that are just huge big rectangles of colour, right? Six! Spread around all over the building. Six!' He waves his arms around and breathes hungrily.

'So they're getting me to do this room, right?' He holds up a finger. 'And I'm going to stick them all in together. All in one room! Next to each other, you know, all together! All those monochrome pictures, all next to each other!' He smiles cheekily, and I smile back: he can tell I think it's the best commentary on modern art I've ever heard. 'It's going to be fucking hilarious! I'll be a made man!'

I start laughing with him. God knows why I'm feeling so happy. He's off the scale and if we don't bring him down he's going to make a serious mess of both our lives.

And this is where it gets sneaky. Because alongside the laughs, I've got an agenda: to make an accurate assessment of him at his worst, and that means whipping him right up into a frenzy. Hang him with his own rope.

'That sounds great,' I say. 'I bet they must be paying you loads, with your talent.'

'Yes! Exactly!' He launches into a full force gale of self-promotion and grandiose flights of fantasy, delighted that I asked, like nobody else wants to listen and I'm the only person who really understands and believes in his inestimable powers – which is kind of almost true. Only he's spent £4,000 in the past week without sleeping a wink, his girlfriend's kicked him out, and it looks like someone punched him square in the face recently.

So I suppose he needs big doses of something to slow him down a bit. More importantly, here we have a very ill man who needs senior input, and my consultant, as ever, is pretending to be at a conference. Doubtless with bathroom sound effects in the background. I call Conrad, my perfect predecessor and trusty saviour.

'No.'

'What?'

'No more informal advice. I want you to phone your consultant, and repeat after me: "Dr Bloch, I feel under-supervised. This is my first job in psychiatry: I need consultant input to manage this patient. It is not safe for me to run a whole clinic on my own."' Oh, Conrad.

'But if I say that, Conrad, he'll give me a bad reference. And then I'll be a failure. For the rest of my life. Stop playing around. Let's botch. It's fine.'

'What do you mean a bad reference? He's a bloody locum. Who cares what he says?'

'What do you mean he's a locum? He's been here for three years. Nobody ever tells me bloody anything.'

'Jesus, Mike. A sixth of all consultant psychiatry posts are unfilled. Nobody wants to do the job anywhere: why should anybody want to do it in this provincial cesspit? Who wants to work in a specialty where you end up feeling responsible for the actions of hundreds of potentially violent and suicidal patients? The money's shit, the service is falling apart and everyone thinks the patients are horrible. We know otherwise of course.'

My patient's great. Oh shit, I left him in the other room!

'Look, Conrad,' I say. 'Just tell me what to do with this guy, OK?'

'OK. Private consultation, Dr Foxton. Keep him in your office.' Sounds good. 'And then while you spend half an hour walking all over the department trying to find your consultant's pager number, he can call his sister in Canada on your mobile, like he did to me last time. *Ker-ching!* One hundred pounds please. Goodbye.'

114

You Don't Have to be Mad to be Here

How low have I sunk as a junior doctor, when I actually look forward to being on-call? Apart from the fact that I secretly love my job, and love the stress, and love being on the spot, and love having a good excuse, now that I'm a psychiatrist, to talk to people about the things that mean most to them: more than that, I love the fact that suddenly there are no machines and communication is my tool.

If that isn't cheesy enough – and I have a big bag of anti-emetics to hand for anyone who appreciated my previous [*cough*] ruggedness – I have a terrible confession to make. In psychiatry, I've found something I'm really bad at. I mean, it's not as if I was ever that good at hospital medicine anyway or I wouldn't be working in this suburban hell-hole.

Anyway, switchboard are very excited because they've just been bought a new pager system that lets them broadcast their voices direct to the little speaker on your bleep, and they can't stop playing with it. Apart from being counter-productive in a psychiatric hospital, this is also rather irritating and weird. The last time I was on-call I woke up the next morning to the sound of the bleeper on the table next to me shouting 'Oi! Take me back to switchboard!' and giggling.

Suddenly it crackles in my pocket. 'Your food's here, Mike. Oh, and there's a 136 on the way.'

These are not two compatible activities. A 136 is someone being brought in on section by the police. I've never seen one, but I've been told they're usually pretty angry. I call the night nurse. Do we accept 136s here?

'Yes, we do,' she sighs in that special way nurses have when faced with yet another junior doctor who will try anything, no matter how pathetic or hackneyed, to avoid doing any more work that involves standing up in their twentieth hour on the go. 'We do accept 136s, Dr Foxton. In the 136 suite. In fact

I can see them driving in right now.'

I look out of the window. So can I. Two police vans. Goodbye curry.

And then all hell breaks loose, or at least that's how it seems to me: somewhere in among the policemen piling in through the door there's some guy who really doesn't want to be here, and there's a lot of shouting, a lot of screaming, a lot of struggling, and a bit of biting.

I stand around and look calm about it, like the nurses. An important policeman comes over.

'Lot of shouting and aggression in a public place. We got called and he went berserk.'

They're holding him down on a foam chair. So far he just looks nasty, not mad.

'Anything odd?' I ask.

The policeman repeats himself, almost word-perfectly. I go over to try and engage my so-called patient.

'Fuck' – he gasps – 'off!' He's wearing seventies Oxfam clothes. Maybe that's why they brought him to me. I try a few more friendly openers.

'Fuck off!'

Still not mad. I try again with the fuzz.

'Did he have anything weird in his pockets?' (Like a note saying *Take me to Dr Foxton. I am quite mad*, maybe?) 'Like a pre-scription, or some tablets? Or an appointment card?' I begin to run out of steam. 'Or, you know, anything, odd . . .'

They look at the man screaming and struggling and then at me, as if the situation should be self-explanatory, which, in a funny way, it should be.

'Look, we've got two-thirds of the county's night-time police force here. Are you going to sedate this bloke so we can get off?' I don't know if you could hear the silent 'or what?' on the end of that sentence.

I look at the patient again and almost will him to do some-thing mad. But he's just angry. I look at the nurses. No back-up.

116

Do they all want to get back to finishing the nightshift paper-work? Or am I actually being an overcautious, sanctimonious twat? I can be a fascist too. I think maybe we should sedate people who behave like this. I don't like them either. But I'm not a policeman, and the rules just aren't like that.

I carry on trying to talk to him and get nothing but sane abuse. The nurses gang up on me.

'We've all got to get back, you know.'

I wish I looked more commanding. I wish I'd worn a better tie. The patient and I both stare at it in a moment of silence. Suddenly he recoils and lets rip.

'The gates! Cambridge! The coat of arms! The twisted staff and snake!'

And out comes the most intensely paranoid delusory system about Cambridge medics that I have ever heard.

Bingo. Haloperidol, 10mg.

Shut-eye and Empathy

I've been on-call for thirty hours so far now. Do you know what that means? Almost solidly awake, mostly on my feet, seeing patients. In fact, seeing vulnerable, sensitive, difficult, sometimes manipulative and often worrying psychiatric patients with com-plicated problems all day, and then all night for emergencies, and then all day again.

Usually you can get a bit of sleep: but you never know and you can never relax, because the bleep is always there, threatening: watching you. This time I was just unlucky. No sleep. A quick lie down. I should be suicidal; and all morning I've had patients complaining of poor sleep. (You drink fifteen cups of coffee a day and you're demanding sleeping tablets.) I dream of sleep, but I'm empathic, and your need is greater than mine. The hours are not going to get to me. I will be nice to the punters. Just as long as I can make it to the canteen and whinge to my mates.

I whinge, and Claire parries (I love her so dearly).

'Have you ever secretly wished that the patient might actually die before you got to casualty,' she asks, 'because you really badly wanted to go to bed?' Everyone giggles.

Aaron blushes. 'I remember when I was a house officer, at 6 a.m., secretly hoping a patient might die on the operating table so I could get to sleep for an hour before the ward round.'

And just for the record – oh eyebrow-raising ones – I can personally guarantee you one thing: these doctors who jokingly admit to nasty feelings like these, they are the ones you would want to be your doctor. Because they're the ones honest enough not to get caught up in that elaborate fantasy doctor world where you're as noble, infallible and omnipotent as the medicine you think you practise. Be human, please.

'So you're coming to the area meeting with the chief exec's office on working hours?'

I smile. Oh yes. So we traipse through to the meetings room, in an immaculately furnished management block, and as the clock ticks through the minutes from the last meeting I imme- diately begin to drop off.

Claire (God, I love her) nobly uses me as an example of how tired a doctor can get.

'Now look, everyone,' the chief executive schmoozes likeably from the white board. 'I hear you have concerns about patient safety.'

Bugger patient safety. When I drive at 5 a.m. across five miles of Home County to see a patient in A&E after a constant trickle of crap calls that stopped me getting any sleep at all so far, what kind of a menace to society am I? Never the best driver, right now my head hurts, my eyes hurt, I'm having difficulty seeing properly and I can't remember which one is the indicator and which one is for the – you know – the things that clean the thing. Oh, hang on. The windscreen wipers. That's it. Sorry, how do I turn them off again? Right.

So then there's all the painful political stuff. I don't even remember it myself. The European Union says we must work no more than forty-eight hours a week by 2009, I think. Until then the trust just incurs ever-higher financial penalties in the form of more money for us. It's called Band III. It has been the cause of some very ugly management bullying in some hospitals, although not here. It's fair, but it depends (ridiculously) on how often you get woken up, on average. It's what we're here for today, to prove we deserve it. That's what they deny.

'Look,' says the chief executive, 'even if you did get Band III, you're going to break the trust's finances, and compromise patient care.'

Swabs please, nurse, to stem this biblical tide of tears. You've known about it for years. Plan ahead. I know these people have a job to do, and I'm sure they're all very nice to their kids. But they can't see that they're chatting casually about whether or not I and all my friends are forced to go through a peculiar form of hell that no one else but a polar explorer would even dream of enduring.

A little empathy, please. A little heart. I look up from my slumber and a spirit of great oratorship strikes me.

'We don't want your money, we want to go to bed.' Eyebrows are raised around the room. 'God. OK. *I* don't want the money.' The chief executive raises his hand in readiness to talk over me. But it's all so wrong. 'Look, I'm a doctor,' I pause for dramatic effect, 'not a fucking stuntman.'

Everyone looks around nervously. The room gradually begins to murmur, then spontaneously erupts into cheers. The chief executive sends us all home early to bed with a pay rise and offers to do Claire's on-call for her this evening so she can go to her sister's birthday party. I wake up. The room is empty.

Pass the Kevlar

Quietly and without fanfare, ambulance crews have started wearing body armour. I stand in the casualty department, staring at them, having a *Daily Mail*-reader moment all on my own. Things in the NHS just aren't what they used to be when I was a fresh-faced new doctor. Two whole years ago.

I've been out in those little vans, prowling the territory, in the dark, in the middle of the night, in those lonely cabs, driving a little bit of hospital around what I now unthinkingly and unpretentiously call 'the community'. And I wet myself even without knowing that there was some rat child out there waiting to stab me.

Now I ask you: who the hell stabs an ambulance man? Who sticks a knife into an ambulance woman? Is it when they're on their way into the building to find the patient or do you wait until they're on their way out, going back to the ambulance? What exactly are you lot playing at out there? It's a wonder we don't drink ourselves to death.

And so to another dinner with the drug reps, another grumpy hangover free of charge. Because there are only about two-and-a-half psychiatrists on the rota here, and I'm the only one who doesn't commute from London, they don't even bother peddling their evil psychiatric drugs on their free nights out. This dinner has been arranged to flog some weird new inhaler to the medics, so they are spared my usual drug-baiting antics.

I wander down to the mess.

'I can't believe you were so rude to that drug rep.'

I casually aim some boiling water at the discount-priced coffee granules and hit a layer of sugar on the work surface as the polystyrene cup flies away. I cough, suavely, as if that was exactly what I meant to do. The two women in the room are pretty attractive, if you go for that haggard-house-officer look. And I'm an SHO now. This is relevant because, as every boy in medicine knows, female doctors only ever snog upwards.

'I mean, I can't believe you were so rude to that drug rep.' I look up innocently, trying to piece together the string of accusations being flung at me by two bionic posh girls watching the football on what is, even by the standards of mess sofas, a very stinky sofa. I breathe my nausea down deeply and cough up some more stale fags.

'Drug reps are there to be baited,' I explain. 'Secretly they like to be kept on their toes.' What could I possibly have had to say about an inhaler? I've been a psychiatrist for five months. I can hardly remember any of that stuff.

'Well, you were doing all right until you told him his flagship antipsychotic was "genius" because the side effects were as bad as all the others but didn't kick in until three months later, by which time you'd already managed to convince the "punters" to take them.'

Sounds perfectly reasonable to me. Actually it sounds rather astute. Make the best of a bad lot and all that.

'And then you started telling him proudly about how you never listen to a word that drug reps say on principle, just after me and Katy convinced him to fund our leaving party.' If this is true I may well be an arse. 'And then you tried to chat up his trainee – who is also his girlfriend. It was, like, so tragic.'

You see? I don't know what's happened to junior doctors. When I was a house officer we used to take bets on which consultant could make the drug reps cry. Now they pander to them. Where's the spirit gone?

I carry my hangover to outpatients for the alcohol clinic – my monthly event where I stick all the biggest boozers in one morning, so that none of my middle-aged depressed housewives complain about the smell – to see Julio, a nurse who has been suspended on full pay in disgrace for six months, with no inquiry, after a sexual-assault allegation was made by a patient who has since retracted all charges. Rather sensibly, he has been drinking three bottles of wine a day since his wife left him. I can't offer him anything that strong.

'What can I do for you, Julio?'

I think it's a good question and I might as well ask him, instead of thinking it over myself.

'Bus pass.'

He's on full pay. It's a meaningless gesture. I fill out the form and lie my arse off, like we always do on DSS forms or they get nothing.

'I'm going to give you post-traumatic stress disorder, with a prominent depressive overlay.'

He smiles. It's the least I can do.

Do Not Interfere with the Fishes

There is a walk of silence of twenty yards from the waiting room to the room where I see patients, and in five months I still haven't worked out how to fill it.

'How's it going?' is clearly wrong, especially for depressed patients. Sometimes I try to make a jovial comment about the fishtank outside the smoking room. Right now there is a man with his sleeves rolled up, fishing in the fishtank.

I wonder if I should say something. A notice next to the aquarium reads: PLEASE DO NOT INTERFERE WITH THE FISHES. I look at Johan, my next punter, feeling like I should know what to do. He leans over to address the fisherman, indicating the staff on the front desk.

'Why don't you go and ask them for some help?' he suggests.

The fisherman nods seriously. 'Yes. Thanks.' He walks off.

'You should change that notice,' Johan says, as aggressive as ever: 'NO MATTER HOW IMPORTANT YOUR MISSION, DO NOT INTERFERE WITH THE FISHES.'

In my first week I thought Johan was trying to kill me. Just goes to show the value of getting to know someone. Sometimes I feel he knows more about schizophrenia than I ever will. What worries me is that he seems to have chosen it as a lifestyle option. We sit down.

'Before you ask,' he says, 'I haven't taken any of your filthy drugs, nor do I plan to, so can we please desist from this farce with the prescription pad at the end?'

Now to an extent, I respect this stance. There is something faintly depressing about depot clinic, where you review all the strangely cowed chronic schizophrenics who have been coming in for their monthly needle for ten years, and sit at home all day smoking for a living.

But it's more complicated than it looks. Those chronic schizophrenics you see on the street doing nothing but smoking and staring: that's not the side effects of the drugs we give them; that's the natural course of the illness. For the most part, they're the ones we missed twenty years ago. That's what I'm trying to avoid with Johan. And he is – although it's a cardinal sin to have one – pretty much my favourite punter.

The longest I've managed to get him taking antipsychotics for is a week, when the voices were getting too much and started to piss him off. I'd also managed to convince him that I could find him a drug that shouldn't make him tired.

'They're shit. They made me sleepy. I flushed them down the toilet.' The game was up. 'Michael, don't expect me to fit into one of your little pigeonholes, because I won't. I'm not mad, and you know you can't section me.'

But I don't want to section him. Well, that's not quite true. The first two times I met him he scared the shit out of me and I whinged to my slack locum consultant down the phone. But Johan presents no real risks, and the worst that can happen is deterioration over the years. And Dr Slack, on his billionaire's locum consultant contract, will do anything to avoid admitting patients to the ward.

'Johan,' I tell him, 'I'm not going to section you. It doesn't matter what you call it: people who hear voices, have delusions, and think MI5 are spying on them (when clearly they're not, by the way) do better on medication in the long run. No matter what you call them.'

'God, you're all so fucking feeble-minded. You just can't cope with anyone who's different. Can you?'

'Look, I'm not your parent or your teacher. There is no gain for me in you taking these drugs. It makes no odds to me either way – it's just you I'm worried about.'

He roars with laughter and gets up. 'One day you'll learn.' And he's gone.

I Should Have Been a Plumber

This week, in 2000, I became a doctor. I've been wiping society's bum for exactly two years. And if it doesn't get better in the next three months, I'm out of the game. Nothing is worth this stress. As Einstein said – except he was talking about the H-bomb – if I'd known then what I know now, I'd have been a plumber.

I went into medicine seven years ago thinking I would be a psychiatrist. Maybe I was just unlucky with this job, but I don't even know if I care any more, because every day it gets worse. I feel like I've been stuck in a room with society's biggest emotional problems with only a couple of textbooks and a prescription pad for support.

The system is so underfunded that there's no way I could ever hope to solve any of my patients' problems, and to get them coping better with what they've got, which I suspect is the idea, I would need to be some kind of miracle worker, or at least a psychiatrist. I'm neither, because nobody has taught me to be, and because I'm just not good enough.

I have this consultant, allegedly, but he is a product of the system too. The job has such a huge workload, and such a burnout rate, that nobody wants to do it, and so the post has been officially empty for years, and filled with temporary locum staff like my boss, and he has no interest in his underlings, and that means me.

So what do I do? I have no one to talk to about patients. I've never seen anyone else seeing a patient outside of video teaching sessions, and all I know is what books tell me.

So here is the paltry sum of my pathetic knowledge of psychiatry, after six months in the game. First, the drugs. If a patient has been well for a longish while, check the calendar, try to reduce the dose and hope nothing goes wrong. If they're not getting better, you increase the dose until you get to the top, and then you change them on to another one, according to side effects. Einstein I am not.

Then we get to the tough stuff. How am I supposed to be? First, I kind of worked out I'm supposed to be a nice person. This may, of course, surprise you. I might seem a bit bullish, because when you're away from it all, and, frankly, you're in a whingy mood, you might tend to revel in your own shit. But these people are fundamentally nice, and have been dealt a string of cruel blows, regardless of whether they're environmental or genetic, and it's impossible not to care.

How nice? Well, that's a good question. Because you're not their friend. You can't be too nice, otherwise they get attached and upset when you go. As I've just discovered. There are some great suggestions in the textbooks. Like getting them to come up with suggestions about what they could do with their problems: because if you make suggestions, they will say no, no, no. But when you lead them into it, with open questions, they own the decision, and they want it. Clever. But it cannot be enough.

The worst thing is: the risks. The suicides. It feels as if it's on my shoulders. I call my boss and tell him about my risk assessments, about my patients who look like they might really do it this time. When I can get hold of him, he says 'Oh dear.' He says nothing. He suggests nothing. He makes me feel more anxious. And I cannot deal with worrying if they'll be alive after the weekend.

It's August. Tomorrow I've got a new job and a new boss. And I give it three months or I'm out. Three months.

I should have been a plumber.

A Textbook Case

I walk into the ward of my new job ten minutes late, with a hangover, to be met by the professor. He grabs my arm.

'Look, if you don't want to iron them, just use a bit more fabric conditioner, leave them to dry in the bathroom, nice bit of steam, let the creases fall out. You wouldn't catch me in a shirt that fucked up, 'cause I'm dapper, you know, I'm the dapper professor, Professor Dap, king of common sense. You're just the doctor, right, maybe, but you've got obligations, now fetch us some more of this terrible food.' This is all, in many ways, fair comment.

Mr Wainwright is a local legend for any junior psychiatrist who has done on-calls in this tedious little town, and he's one reason I was pleased to get my job. He cycles into mania faster than anyone I know, but he knows exactly what's going on because he was in my new boss's study on patient education and knows more about manic depression than any doctor.

The first time I met him was in A&E at 3 a.m., when he counted up his symptoms on a piece of paper and wrote exactly how much medication he thought he was going to need to come down. Most doctors feel slightly anxious about this kind of thing, especially because people always like being manic. Maybe it feels like a pay-off for the depressive phases: a part of them wants to stay up there. But this man knew his last three lithium levels and had a written list of his previous admissions. Money can't buy the love that brings at 3 a.m.

I excuse myself (and there is no greater test of your cocktail party skills than disengaging from a manic patient) and make my way to the nursing station for a first impression. There are a lot of pitfalls that junior doctors can fall into with nurses, but the textbook classic is that they decide you're a snotty, work-shy ex-public schoolboy who thinks he's better than God. In psychiatry, the nurses know the patients better than anyone. So you really don't want to give them that idea.

Before I get two paces I am headed off.

'New doctor?'

I prepare my helpful smile.

'Patient short of breath in the clinic room.'

I chose psychiatry so I could leave that kind of thing behind. I don't want to work. I've got a hangover. The nurse points down the corridor and we trot (running? In psychiatry?) to the clinic room, where there is the sickest looking patient I have seen in six months. She's in a psychiatric hospital for anxiety and she's short of breath. I'm suspicious. I put on my I-understand-but-I-am-not-going-to-conspire-with-hypochondriacal-pathology face and hope there's nothing wrong with her. Her pulse is 105: she has a swollen calf and chest pain. And with the £2.50 stethoscope from the ward – while making a mental note to carry a proper stethoscope in future – I swear I can hear creaking leather.

You don't often hear creaking leather with a pulmonary embolism, although it's *the* textbook sign of it. And I dimly recall that they can be rather dangerous. I call the nearest proper hospital and am met with every junior psychiatrist's nemesis: the sarcastic medical registrar.

I tell him I think I have a PE.

'What makes you think that?'

'I can hear creaking leather.'

'Creaking leather? Like in the textbooks?'

'Like in the textbooks.'

'That's good. I've never heard creaking leather like in the textbooks.'

'Well, no. Neither had I until today.'

'Well, I suppose I'd better take it then.'

'Is that OK?'

'Oh God, it's fine. Anything else over there? Perhaps you've spotted some Roth's Spots and diagnosed SBE?'

I put down the phone politely. So nurses think all doctors are arseholes? I take a breath and prepare to start again with my cheesy smile.

Flying Doctor

'Is there a doctor on the flight?'

I look up surreptitiously. Episodes like this dredge up all kinds of ugly feelings in any doctor. It's a cracking opportunity to be a bit of a hero, which we like – and there must be plenty of attractive and single air stewardesses out there. But most doctors, since we're mostly NHS and not privately insured, think twice before helping strangers nowadays. We've all heard the stories about a friend of a friend who got sued over a minor cock-up in the process of saving a life.

You see, if you're nasty to us, I'm afraid we stop being nice to you. We're too human and too underpaid to subsidize your bad spirit. A nation recoils in indignation. Aren't you obliged to help? What – and get sued? Frankly, no.

So I sit there for ten seconds, seething self-righteously.

'Is there a doctor on the flight?'

There's nothing different or special about being a doctor, you know. Plenty of other professions are in a position to relieve the pain of strangers, they just choose not to. Like the person who sits on the check-in desk at the airport who very nearly buggered my holiday – whose job it is to say things like 'I'm sorry, sir: check-in for that flight closed two minutes ago'; who can listen to a distressed, sleep-deprived junior doctor saying 'But please, you've got to help me: if I don't get on that plane I will lose my girlfriend/only holiday this year' and really mean it – and who didn't care.

The person who does that job has the power to go the extra mile, fix problems, alleviate pain and prevent real, serious damage to people's lives.

No, it is not different. It is the same.

I straighten my shirt and stand up, smiling.

The stewardess heads me off with the medical box and retreats. I take a peek. It has lots of exciting-looking stuff in it, but none of those nice pocket-sized medical textbooks we occasionally (*coughs*) like to refer to. That's fine. The patient's probably just had a heart attack. I catch myself hoping that the bag doesn't have anything too complicated, like IV atropine or a central line.

I look over the patient. He doesn't seem to be in pain. In fact, he's not moving at all. I touch him: he's cold. He is, on cursory inspection, dead.

At this point, I'd like to make clear that, belligerent though I may often appear, in the flesh I am always nice and polite; and, despite my private rant, it took me fifteen seconds to get here from the time the announcement was made. Human bodies, I would guess, must have similar heat-retaining properties to the average central-heating radiator: they couldn't have got him this cold in less than a quarter of an hour.

I listen to his chest with a stethoscope and all I hear is very loud engine noise.

Poor bloke. And he was alone. So I certify him and scribble some basic medical notes. And then they bring me three more forms. I spend my whole life filling in forms. I was happy to work for free, but there's no way I'm signing those forms, on principle. I only came to help out. I didn't do anything as a doctor. He was already dead.

I look at the forms. They are covered in legal words, not medical ones. They speak of 'liability'.

'What about my forms?' I want to say, and not for the first time. 'Fill out this fucker. Yes, your National Insurance number and your paternal grandmother's maiden name. Well, I'm sorry, I can't help you unless you do.'

I hedge and look baffled: I just helped you out with this guy out of the kindness of my heart.

They are very insistent, almost threatening. Everyone is watching. I feel like the in-flight entertainment.

So I sign the forms and I sit down again and seethe until we land. As I get off the plane, the stewardess presses a gift bag into my hand. It contains six laminated drinks coasters and a plastic model of an aeroplane. So it looks as if you and I both get exactly what we deserve.

What a Team

'Is it safe for Mr Hunter go to the drop-in centre unaccompanied?'

Mr Hunter is very nice and extremely depressed. It looks like a simple enough question, but about ten times a day I'm expected to be a soothsayer. I think briefly about patting my pockets and making a lame joke about leaving my crystal ball at home, before I remember my new resolution not to be fatuous at work.

So this is the deal. We are employed, among other things, to assess risk, a job that no one can ever do perfectly – and you lot are obsessed with it, to the detriment of patient care. If we get the answer wrong and something terrible happens, you read about it in the newspapers and we get hauled up for a bit more public hatred. Or alternatively, if we keep everyone in, you think we're all sinister control freaks who like locking up people for our own rather expensive amusement and self-justification. It is, as you can see, a fine line.

The staff are looking at me and I feel obliged to give a definite answer. A definite answer will assuage the anxiety on the ward by passing it on to me (in exchange for cash at the end of the month) and make everyone feel like everything is under control. A definite answer will make people think that I am a confident, sensible, efficient and helpful young psychiatrist. A definite answer would also be a lie. It would perpetuate the myth that it is possible to give definite answers about this kind of thing.

Once again, I am at the same crossroads in life: facile self-aggrandizement and maintaining the hegemony in one direction, or an act of honest weakness and shoulder-shrugging that would – should it become a regular pattern – torpedo my career. It's biblical stuff going on here, I'm telling you.

I have a quick look through the notes. Questions about risk have been an ugly blind spot for me, because my last boss so expertly avoided it that I used to feel as if it was all my problem – which at the time, of course, it was.

A flashback: Dr Foxton, in his first week as a psychiatrist, asking his consultant if a risky patient hinting at suicide should come to the hospital.

'Well, it's difficult, isn't it? It depends on so many factors.' I know. I've told you about them. Yes or no would do. 'I remember a patient I had once . . .' I know. Back in 'Nam, perhaps? Yes or no, please. 'Of course, it never used to be like this, you know, before they closed the old sanatoriums. Anybody risky was just kept in.' I know. You told me. Hands up. Yes or no? Please. Or I'll shoot.

I shudder and remember where I am. It's OK. I have a new boss. I can see his reassuring handwriting in the notes. What would he do? At this point he ambles in. A boss who is willing to share responsibilities for his patients is one thing, but a psychic is beyond my wildest dreams. Perhaps he can tell me what the patient is thinking.

I ask him if it's OK for Mr Hunter to go to the drop-in centre alone. He smiles warmly and turns to the nurse who asked me.

'What do you think, Bill?'

It's genius. Why didn't I think of that? And then we all agree that, yes, Mr Hunter can go to the community centre alone.

Did you hear that? We all agree. We all seamlessly pooled our expertise. Picture the scene at the coroner's inquest; picture that weighing light on our consciences if everything goes pear-shaped. It's like those psychology experiments on shameless Nazi prison guards where they all thought it was someone else's responsibility. Only much nicer. Shared responsibility feels so good. Even if it goes horribly wrong, it can't feel too bad.

I drag myself back from my reverie and get up to catch my consultant at the door.

'You remember Kirsty Farmer who went home last weekend?'

'Oh yes, nice girl, horribly depressed. Taken an overdose, has she?' he asks in the warmest, most welcoming tones imaginable, as if taking an overdose would have been a manageable outcome of her going home (on my recommendation); a problem, very sad, but nobody's fault, another situation to deal with.

'No,' I say, wiped out by this response. 'She has come back to collect her things. She sends her regards.'

'That's nice. Do send her mine.' And he's off. Back to heaven, perhaps. Or to the orphanage to distribute toys to the poor.

Time for a Happy Meal

'I'm still depressed. I'm not getting better. You're a useless doctor and this clinic is a farce. I'm writing a letter of complaint.'

I smile warmly.

'And what the hell are you smiling about? My wife says I'm suicidal and it'll be on your head.'

This nasty scene raises interesting problems. First, it is quite possible I'm a useless doctor, though I'm not sure how you'd measure that. In general medicine, when a little old lady is grateful for your help getting over pneumonia, you know where you stand. In psychiatry it's more dangerous: you can't derive your sense of how well you're doing from how much the patients like you.

For example, in this morning's clinic, if I had prescribed the lifetime supply of Valium that one person was demanding, they'd probably be writing to their MP as we speak, recommending me for a knighthood. I could have exaggerated another person's illness on a form to the council and got them one step closer to a bigger council house. I could have conspired with a hypochondriac and ordered them a whole pile of hospital tests.

Actually, on reflection, I can't be bothered to lie to you. I did both of those last two things. But I was trying really hard not to.

Oh God. I'm a terrible doctor. This patient really hates me. And I'm not even professional enough to help him take responsibility for his feelings. The way he's staring at me, I can't think of a word to say. I can't see how he could ever get better. Even I think it's my fault this man is depressed. And I can never remember the side effects of Quaxipram.

Oh God. I bet they all commit suicide before the weekend. My consultant will sack me and they'll put my photograph and my parents' home phone number on the front cover of the local paper.

And suddenly here I am, eating a Happy Meal with my new consultant. You maybe don't know how odd that is, so you'll have to take my word for it.

'Of course, my wife is an orthopod,' he says. 'She thinks anything other than surgery is a waste of a medical degree.' He smiles warmly. An orthopod, incidentally, is an orthopaedic surgeon: they're usually very male and their hobbies include assuming traditional gender roles. At parties, when they meet psychiatrists, they shout things like 'only steel can heal' before quaffing more beer and becoming sexually inappropriate.

And then we talk about my patient.

'Sometimes, you know, when people make you feel like that, especially if they're blaming you for everything, they might have some' – he looks out of the window – 'some quite maladaptive personality traits.'

He says it so neutrally, like it's all just part of the clinical problem. Like no one is at fault. Which, of course, I knew all along. Which is, of course, part of the job. I just forgot somehow, stuck in the clinic room with those toxic stares.

'It might be a long run getting him to deal better with life. We could talk about how you could approach it, if you like. Are you seeing him some time next month?'

I look at the floor. I was so freaked out I made an appointment to see him later this week. This is not boundaried time-management. I ask what will happen when he complains.

My consultant smiles and sips his coffee. 'You'll be ever so slightly demoralized. I'll have to stay late to go through the notes, and lesser doctors would think about leaving the profession.' He pushes his glasses up his nose and smiles. I want to be that man.

I Don't Want Your Money

'The NHS is over; we're all going to be rich. They've really pissed on their chips this time.'

My registrar is in a particularly bad mood: he has just seen the Health Minister on TV accusing doctors of being greedy for not accepting the new consultants' contract.

I look around the drab on-call room. It's not easy doing a day's work, working the whole night and then working the whole of the next day. Working thirty-three hours in a row makes you feel shit: it makes you split up with your girlfriend, it loses you your mates, it stops you going out and it makes you crap at your job. It's illegal, except that the Government got some special dispensation to exempt us from EU employment law. And it's cruel. You just need more doctors. So train more doctors.

So why have we always done it? Not for the money: my basic salary is £24,000 and I'll send you a photocopy of my payslip to prove it. We do it because we have a collective Mother Teresa complex and, to be honest, because it feels good to work insanely hard, but to know that you are doing a good job for society, and that you are appreciated for it.

But when people start to be rude about us on telly, when we are all made to look like the minority who practise badly, when patients are over-demanding and rude to us in casualty and in GP surgeries, then that's it. I'm telling you, with the mood every doctor in the country is in, this is the end of the NHS, the greatest state healthcare system in the world, which we were all truly proud to work in.

And get this: with the attacks on doctors in the media, and patients' temper tantrums in casualty at three in the morning, the NHS will be killed for ever, not by some restructuring or government policy, but by sheer, simple, old-fashioned rudeness. It's not ironic, it's stupid and sad.

So this is what happened with the new contract. We are not greedy. We did not go to the Government demanding more money. They came to us and told us we had to stop doing private practice, and be available to work until 10 p.m. and over the whole weekend for the entirety of our working lives, until we retire, in exchange for a bit more money. Needless to say we prescribed the big Fuck Off tablet. You would too.

In one hospital where I used to work, the surgeons say they are all going to leave the NHS, *en masse*, and set up private chambers like lawyers. And you know how expensive lawyers are. I've never heard doctors talk like this before. The irony is, these are people who used to stay late every day, working way beyond their contracts out of a sense of duty to the country and their patients. That's over. Applications to medical school are down for the first time and doctors are haemorrhaging out of the profession to do other jobs.

Now I don't blame patients for being rude sometimes. I've had patients threaten to hit me because they've been kept waiting in A&E. I've had patients pull out video cameras to film my explanation of why the consultant is too busy to come and personally give the explanation for an operation (he was in the theatre battling against waiting lists). I know it can be frightening to wait in casualty, because I've done it. I know it's irritating to wait two weeks for an appointment. And for years you've been made to feel like consumers instead of citizens, so you are going to be demanding. But people have got to be civil. It is not the doctors' fault. And we're human too.

Hospitals in big cities, especially London, have huge nursing bills now, because the wages were so unworkably low for so long that half of the NHS nurses left and were replaced by agency staff on twice the money. Your money. In many parts of the country, in some specialties, consultant posts are empty: because it is a great job, but it is a difficult job, and it looks like nobody wants to do it for the money being offered.

Those empty posts are filled with agency doctors, and they get £180,000 a year. Which is what doctors get in Europe; you don't even want to think about doctors' bills in the United States. You could have had doctors for a quarter of that. We didn't ask for the money. But it looks as if £180,000 is the going rate for the job since we started being attacked on TV. I hope you all enjoy paying it as much as we will enjoy spending it. Bring it on, Alan Milburn.

It's OK to Have Feelings, Isn't It?

So it's 3 a.m. and I get called to the ward.

Ha! Fooled you. Actually it's 10 p.m., so I'm far from grumpy. Actually, I'm in rather a good mood. I trundle over to the ward, all smiles. The nurses look worried.

'We need you to rewrite some PRN.'

Now, PRN are tablets that the nurses dish out when they need to. Rewriting it is often a source of tedious friction. Doctors on-call get miffed about doing it at night, when the chart runs out of spaces, because really that sort of thing should get sorted during the day. I understand that to you that seems really boring and petty. To us it is the difference between sleeping and not. Remember, they use sleep deprivation to torture people very effectively in some places. So now you know. But I'm far from miffed. I'm in a good mood. It's only 10 p.m.

'Thanks doctor, he's really distressed and just needs some more lorazepam.'

Now, watch how I make all kinds of unnecessary trouble for myself. Normally, you just rewrite the chart and do a runner. But remember it's only 10 p.m. and for some reason I'm in the mood to be a proper psychiatrist.

'Does he really need it?' I ask.

Everyone looks at me suspiciously. I mean, people come into hospital depressed, usually because they present a suicide risk or we need to tinker with complicated medication. But it's OK to have feelings. Even bad ones. Admitting someone to a psychiatric ward and filling them up with drugs to stop them feeling anything, that's the oldest cliché in the book. We don't do things like that any more unless we have to.

I grab the notes, with the uncomfortable feeling that people are starting to think I'm questioning their professional judgement. In many ways, psychiatric nurses are amazing. They work in the same place for years, unlike a lot of medical wards that are full of agency staff, and they always know the patients better than you. You could go through the whole of your career doing exactly what they tell you to do and everything would be fine.

But lorazepam is the same as mother's little helpers. It's a benzo; a nice warm feeling in a pill. It's an easy way to make things manageable for everyone in the short term. It's like drinking. It's too easy. In a parallel universe I would have swallowed a textbook and be standing here shamelessly in front of you, talking about how it is an institutionalized maladaptive coping strategy.

They point out of the window at a man who is utterly – and I mean utterly – distraught. We have a quick chat and he is painfully, gut-wrenchingly unhappy. My first impulse is to do anything I humanly can to make it stop. I look back at the notes. Nowhere does it say that part of their plan is to repress all emotions with benzos. But it wouldn't, would it? These things just develop gradually. It would be an easy thing to miss. And looking at the chart, it only ever happens at night, when there are always different staff on. And the doctors' signatures on the chart are all different, so they're probably duty doctors too.

I look up. Everyone is baffled that I haven't just rewritten it and buggered off, including me. Who do I think I am? Some junior doctor who was working in A&E nine months ago. It is the easiest thing in the world to rewrite it.

I think back to this afternoon and our History of Psychiatry teaching. You know, thirty years ago, when we were just starting to get a handle on drugs for psychiatric problems, we were dishing out these tablets called Dexamyl – half-amphetamine and half-barbiturates – like they were Smarties. 'The antidepressant that works in an hour' was the strapline. I can think of plenty of street dealers who would happily provide a similar service.

What a drug: but more than that, how great it must have felt, as a doctor, to be presented with distressed, depressed patients and for it to feel like the best and most natural thing in the world to give them a mixture of uppers and downers, and make it all go away. Imagine how grateful the patients must have been. Imagine not thinking there was anything wrong with it.

I look at the chart. I look at the nurses. I take a long look at the patient. And I find myself rewriting the chart, looking at no one, and mumble something I hope is helpful, about maybe trying to avoid giving them out too often. And while I scribble something quickly in the notes, I wonder what it would be like to be good at my job, and how I'd ever know if I was.

Never Again

So there I am, picking pubic hairs off the soap in the doctors' on-call shower, when suddenly the immense historical significance of this moment strikes me: tomorrow all the rotas in the hospital change. Tomorrow the trust becomes New Deal-compliant. And tonight we will be the last doctors in this hospital ever to work thirty-three hours in a row. If I hadn't been in the shower, you might have caught a fond tear of remembrance falling from the corner of my eye.

I went to the doctors' mess and announced the significance of this moment, and we wept for lost friends. I remember so well, during a night on-call with not a jot of sleep, how Phoebe slipped on the stairs on the way to an arrest bleep and ended up with her leg in a cast for six weeks. The nurses wrote *RoboDoc* on the back of her white coat. How we laughed.

Waites remembered how his girlfriend would playfully bottle up all the frustration of nights without him, and engage him in lovers' tiffs we could all hear from the other end of the accommodation block as he wept and begged for sleep. How we all smiled.

You cannot even begin to imagine what sleep deprivation on that scale is really like, and I can hardly imagine it being over. There are moments of horrible madness and desperation. I keep quiet, for example, about the awful lonely moment I thought I might actually be losing my mind – no sleep for fifty hours, walking through empty hospital corridors, with my nerves buzzing, these fine vibrations in my perception, as if the whole world was shimmering backwards and forwards, and the sound of 'I Could Have Danced All Night' from *My Fair Lady* blasting just a little bit too loud in my head.

But now it's gone. No more will I stand by the roll-up doors at 4 a.m., where the *Moonraker* buggies with the meals and the linen go into the hospital basement, smoking a cigarette and pretending I'm James Bond.

It's a con, of course.

They are taking us off an on-call rota – where we work all day, all night, and then all of the next night – and putting us on weeks of nights and extended days until 9 p.m. But there are no more doctors and there is still just as much work to be done, and the total hours don't change: it's just rejigged so that we do shorter on-calls more frequently. Just like before, if you add up the number of extra days and hours we do, because you don't get a day off in the week to compensate, it's roughly the same over a year as if we did a normal job, but with no holiday, ever. The only thing that's changed is the extreme sports sleep-deprivation stuff.

Please just employ more doctors. It's very simple.

So anyway, as is traditional after a night on-call, I drive home to have dinner with my parents, whom I adore most at my weakest moments, and announce this historic moment to my dad. He sniffs over the peas.

'When I were a lad, we used to do a one in two on-call, up every other night. And we used to sleep at t'bottom of t'sharps bin and be glad of it.'

My mum looks up. 'Well, it was kind of different then, dear. Do you remember how I used to hide under the duvet when the porters brought you your cup of tea in the morning?'

Tea in bed on-call? We're lucky if they keep the canteen open after eight.

'And remember how angry you were that morning, when you realized you'd forgotten to leave your shoes outside the door to be polished?'

And then it all comes out. They had silver service. Really, properly: dinner on-call was laid out in the doctors' mess on silver trays. And my dad's not that old. They would hang out in the on-call room playing pool. Occasionally a nurse would call them to the wards, where they would have laid out the notes, and the drug charts that needed doing, ready for you when you got there. And when someone had a cardiac arrest, well, there wasn't much you could do about it anyway. You would just think 'Oh dear,' jot something in the notes, and potter off back to bed.

Now I'm not asking for anyone to bow down to me, because it's weird and gross and wrong. But at least then they were looked after. So please, just please employ more doctors, try and be civil, and give me back my life.

Foreign Nurses for Christmas

Christmas is a time of guilt. So here I am, putting up the Christmas decorations, cleaning my stinky sock of a flat, and having yet another extended Residents' Association debate over the Jif about whether or not it's acceptable to employ a cleaner just because you are a junior doctor, when suddenly I realize the moment has arrived.

Today I must finally confront the three-foot pile of unopened copies of the *British Medical Journal*, which has been mocking me from the corner of the sitting room since the day I moved in a year ago.

Why did I even bring them with me? I know I'm never going to read them. Normally I try not to do myself out of a column by dealing with issues only doctors will understand, but the *BMJ* comes free to every doctor in the country and I think, secretly, all of you girls and boys, if you'd just look into your hearts and confront your demons: you know you'll never even open them. It's not that we don't want to read about 'Prevalence of gastroschisis at birth: a retrospective cohort study', but there must be an impoverished library somewhere that could put them to much better use.

Anyway, I'm not a bad person. Sometimes I read the useful bits on-line to calm down after I realize that my ex really isn't going to e-mail me and is probably having sex with some muscular pop star.

So my Christmas present to the world today is to take each and every one of these *BMJ*s out of their plastic wrappers – it's going to take hours – and find a good way of recycling them.

Our hospital, on the other hand, has received a wonderful Christmas gift from Sri Lanka this week: thirty-five new nurses for the surgical wards. I think, in a lot of ways, even from a non-Christian country, this exemplifies gloriously the giving spirit of Christmas: those who can ill afford to give coming together to give us something we don't really need.

I've worked for years in hospitals full of nurses that we've plundered from the Third World, and they're great. I mean, they are really great nurses (because most nurses are) and they work hard for really low wages, the kind of wages British people quite rightly turn up their noses at, and so in that sense we kind of do need them.

And a darker part of me even thinks that maybe it was good for the fair few racist little old ladies and gentlemen that I've dealt with on general medical wards to have to confront their latent fascist views, in their twilight minutes, as they edged their way towards their final judgement day, on the off-chance that God turns out to be a *Guardian* reader.

But nurses are a natural resource. They are dug like gems from the dry earth and nurtured rather expensively by state-funded training programmes. In the countries we plunder our nurses from they don't have a lot of money to squander. And so it really is very Christmas-spirited of these struggling nations to hand over their nurses – after a little prompting from the two ward managers who nobly went out for two weeks in the summer recruiting them.

I digress. You see, I never would have noticed if I hadn't gone out Christmas drinking with the surgeons last night after their exams, and heard them grumbling, as they all start to apply for registrar jobs, about how all their prized positions are being taken by doctors from Asia who will all go back to their own countries in five years' time after being fully trained up here, and moaning about crap referrals from locum GPs who have only just arrived in the country and can't speak English very well, who are all working in inner-city practices where no doctor in their right mind would volunteer to work.

Now I wouldn't want you to think that surgeons are all about racism and tit jokes, and to be fair most of the evening was spent talking about NHS trusts being sued by the partners of people who had metal staple repairs to their haemorrhoids and didn't think the issue through before they had anal sex. (Apparently it's like grinding your penis on to a cheese grater covered in poo.)

But as my gift to the world [*nobly places hand on heart*] I'm going to find a way to send my embarrassing, unread *BMJ*s to doctors in the developing world. Maybe. And in the meantime, maybe you could all sort out a government that treats doctors and nurses a bit more civilly, so that we wouldn't need to go around stealing them from people who need them far more than we do at Christmas.

The Horrors of Tribunals

'You're a shit doctor who never listens and I'll be out of here by lunchtime.'

I had almost forgotten it was Nigel's tribunal. We were getting on pretty well until today, but I guess his solicitor has been talking to him. That means we won't be friends for a while and he'll be refusing his medication for at least a week. I try and smile warmly until I remember how paranoid it makes him.

I hate sectioning people. Nigel had to be sectioned because he was going around telling everyone in his council block that they should stop selling crack to their children. He didn't start getting beaten up until he suggested to the parents that they should hand the children over into his care, where he could give them the love they needed. It was all very well meant, but you just have to try and work around the fact that people get angry about that kind of thing in the middle of the night.

We all trundle through the corridors to the conference room. Nigel stands, with his solicitor, staring at me. I stand with the nurse and the social worker. The tribunal keeps us waiting for half an hour, until we are called in by the clerk.

They all have cups of coffee and neat little china plates with biscuits on them. The barrister who is chairing the hearing addresses everyone by their formal title, and we sit on opposite sides of the table: everyone has an expensive leather documents folder and a suit, except for me and Nigel. I feel deeply out of place, and very worried.

'Dr Foxton, are you satisfied that the patient has a mental illness, disorder, or impairment; and that it is of a nature and degree such as to justify detention under the Mental Health Act 1983?'

Umm.

'Yes,' I reply, confidently.

'Yes, what?'

I look around. 'Yes, your honour?' I smile weakly and start to sweat. Taking off my jumper now would look really bad.

The tribunal doctor looks over warmly. He is about seventy, clearly retired, and being paid by the hour. 'When the chair asks you that question, he means: which of the three is it, under the terms of the Mental Health Act? Is it nature or degree or both?' I look up at him, willing him to help me out some more. 'You have to say which, now.'

The chair casts him an evil look. He smiles back.

'Umm. Illness,' I flounder. 'And, well, nature and degree, please.'

I had never really thought about it. I blush again.

Nigel looks baffled and delighted. The barrister just looks angry and rich.

Nigel's solicitor rounds on me and makes me go through my report. I have to recount, in front of Nigel, all of his psychiatric symptoms in the most technical medical language, because this is a formal legal hearing.

It feels as if I'm accusing him of a crime: you are charged with stopping taking your medication at home, and hearing voices, and that those voices did compel you to behave very strangely; you are charged with getting into a squabble on a crowded ward with a nasty character over cigarettes, where your understandable misunderstanding of her mental health problems led you to get into a nasty argument and to you both being sedated and secluded.

It would feel massively trite and completely counter-productive to mention that Nigel is incredibly charming and funny, and that his delusions and hallucinations are so painfully understandable, in the context of his shit life, that you sometimes feel like giving him a big hug and trying to explain it all as best you can. Either way, after I read out the list of charges he will probably never tell me about a single symptom ever again for as long as he lives.

Nigel keeps interrupting to deny these episodes. His solicitor pulls my report apart, implying that I am some kind of sinister jailer.

I think back to our teaching: tribunals are supposed to be inquisitorial, not adversarial. We are supposed to get together and work out what's best for the patient. But these guys all want to be on *Judge Judy*. They grill me for an hour, even though there is no way in a million years anyone would let Nigel out of hospital until the medication starts to kick in and gets him back to his normal self. When we start discussing his insight, I deliver what now feels like my trump card – and I realize I have sunk to their level.

'He told me yesterday that if he got off at the tribunal he would leave hospital immediately and stop taking the tablets.' QED.

'I never!' shouts Nigel.

The tribunal retires to consider. But everyone knew the verdict before we even started. The lawyers are a few pounds richer and a few inches taller; and Nigel and I will have to start all over again from square one.

Sometimes It Pays to Keep Mum

'I just, you know, can't really see the point, doc, you know?'

I know how he feels. I think I'm losing my faith in psychiatry – especially with depressed people. Because today, apart from the drugs (and they do work, so don't even try to take that away from me), it seems like it's all theatre, and I hate the theatre.

There's this guy I see every month. Like most inexperienced psychiatrists, I see my depressed patients more frequently than I need to, mainly because of a magical belief that this will prevent them from killing themselves. But this guy thinks he's missing something: and I wonder sometimes if he is really depressed. His life, to be fair, is pretty miserable.

We have a thing called the bio-psycho-social model, which we all buy into. The bio bit is drugs. The social bit is changing the concrete stuff in your life, and that usually means firing off a few letters for the benefits agency to ignore.

But the psychological stuff: this might come as a shock, but nobody really teaches you much about it very quickly. You get a bit about how to listen to people, but psychoanalysts we are not, and really it's like anything in medicine, you just pile in and have a go. I guess it comes with time.

So a few months ago with this guy, I found myself thinking: I completely buy into the idea that people buy the stuff they see on TV to make themselves feel better; but maybe it goes deeper than that. Maybe all the happy people on telly make folk think they ought to be a bit happier than they can ever hope to be. It's like all those worries people had about novels a hundred years ago: you wouldn't want the servants reading them, in case they started getting funny ideas.

I wanted to tell him all this, but obviously I didn't. What I did was – in my own flaky way – try to show him how people can learn coping strategies and be as happy as they can manage. I also wanted to maybe, you know, recommend some improving literature. Which obviously I also didn't do. The worst thing was, because I like him and because he is a bit like my friends, I wanted to tell him about stuff, maybe show him that my life was a bit crap too. It would have been vastly inappropriate, of course, because depression is irrational, and because he is feeling real pain to an extent that I don't: but I challenge you to show me a psychiatrist alive who hasn't had the same thought flicker across their mind at least once.

I'm so glad I didn't. Because today, after six months of seeing me, and after three years of seeing psychiatrists, he decides to tell me something he has never told anyone: his uncle used to fiddle with him. He giggles, and then he won't even look at me.

His uncle didn't used to fiddle with him: he used to take him into a room, pull down his trousers and do unspeakable, horrific things to him. Things that he couldn't tell his wife about or his friends – and he has good friends – or his doctors.

And it wasn't because I am any good as a psychiatrist – I'm not. It was partly time, and it was partly because I never told him about my life or my friends or my favourite bands. To him I'm just a guy in a room who tells him about the side effects of Quaxipram and listens while he talks. To him, I'm a blank slate. He didn't want my approval or respect, so he could tell me anything, and finally he told me everything.

It was only a start, but at last I can understand why we have ground rules about not talking about ourselves, and also why psychiatry can do some small good: maybe the drugs were just a good excuse for two people to sit in a room talking without it having to be called therapy. Now tell me what to do with the other nine people I'm seeing today.

An Enemy for Life

Here we are again, working away at the coalface of human misery with a teaspoon. We all move jobs every six months, in

February and August. Another job, another set of nutters to work with – and a new set of patients. (That's my really funny joke about mental-health workers.)

I immediately spot that I've been shafted by my predecessor in my first morning's clinic when I see a set of five social problems in a row. One is a new patient follow-up. The handover plan says *refer to community team* and I couldn't agree more. Unhappy mother, no money, no friends, no hope, depressed, reasonably suicidal. I potter down the corridor to see the social-work manager and make a referral.

'So what exactly do you want us to achieve, Mike?' she asks. It's a fantastic question: goal-directed and focused, multi-disciplinary work at its best. I ponder the answer to this excellent question. I flounder. Of course, we both know that the answer is this: 'Umm, spend a bit of time with her, do a couple of visits, you know, reach out, make friends, offer a bit of nonspecific support and hope she doesn't kill herself in the meantime.' She looks at me as if she is equally pondering the suggestion that she eat her own poo.

'Well, I don't really see what we can offer her as a team, over what you're doing in your outpatients appointments.' She's getting weirdly angry.

Now the response to this is clear: doctors have a caseload five times that of community nurses and social workers, so we can't see people as often. That's just the way it is. I've been in this job for three hours. This is not the time to start a fight with an assertive social worker twice my age.

I gently try to push my case. She pushes back: she gets (and I mean this) *seriously* aggressive. It's easy to forget that people can, sometimes, use the implication that they might actually twat you to great effect in the workplace. I'm scared. I push harder. This has never happened to me before. I'm not asking her to deskill her staff. The patient just needs a bit of nonspecific support. She starts shouting.

I retreat to my room for a think. I've got six months in this place. There's a blank page in the notes. The patient has gone, with a four-week follow-up appointment. I look at the empty page with my pen in my hand. There's this vague idea going around among doctors that you should always picture yourself in the coroner's inquest when you write your notes.

'Dr Foxton, you were the last doctor to see this patient before she killed herself.' The judge looks down his glasses at me across his nose, as I fill my trousers. 'Your notes read as follows: *Impression: severe depressive episode plus social problems. Plan: refer to social worker.*' He frowns and looks back at my notes. 'You then continue: *Outcome: social worker shouted at me. I realized that I had to work in this place for six months and she scared me. I'm only little and I look about nineteen. I realized that I did not have the social skills to deal with the situation and retreated to my room in search of an easy life. Impression: I am flaky and weak. Too embarrassed to telephone and offer patient follow-up any sooner. Plan: review in four weeks. Work on assertiveness skills. Hope patient not dead by then.*'

I'm sure they're overstretched. Maybe she's had bad experiences with poncy doctors in the past. I've got on all right with social workers everywhere else I've worked. Maybe I should have buttered her up with a bit of chat about public-sector pay and the war in Iraq first. I phone the patient and ask her to come back in a week. It looks like I'll be filling out the benefits forms and talking to the school myself. I'd rather drink bleach than try to refer to the social workers again. Who cares about going home before seven? I'm twenty-six. Stroll on retirement.

I'd Rather Section Myself

I really hate sectioning people.

'No! Please don't! Please! I just want to go home and be with my daughter.'

Oh Christ, when people beg and plead. I don't have the stomach to be a jailer. Now I don't want to present this as a

horror story. It's definitely the right thing to do: this girl is horribly vulnerable to exploitation and there are candidates lining
up for the job out there who are well documented in the notes.
And she only wants to go home because of some awful delusion
about what is going to happen to her on the ward. But however
I sell it to myself, there is still an innocent-looking girl in front
of me who is terrified, and she is terrified of what I'm going to
do to her. This is not a junior doctor feel-good moment.

I sit down, tired and wired by the whole experience, fill out
the form in a hurry and hand it to the nurse in charge. He snig-
gers.

'According to this form, in your professional opinion you have
grounds to detain Dr Michael Foxton under section 5(2) of the
Mental Health Act 1983.'

Sectioning myself, in many ways, would be the neatest way
out of this ugly episode. I tear up the form in a hurry and write
out another. There can't be many junior doctors on-call who
haven't at least toyed with the idea of admitting themselves for a
bit of a rest.

Then I think: I know what I'd want if I were this deluded and
frightened and vulnerable. I'd want to be sectioned. Hands
down, no question about it. And the drugs, too, however imper-
fect they might be. Although I might want a veto on a few of
them. I would even have ECT as a last resort, honestly: because
I know it is safe and I have seen it work.

Right. Look. There are three reasons to section somebody:
(1) risk to self, (2) risk to others and (3) risk of deterioration. If,
one day, I'm scared and confused and a danger to others (which
this girl isn't, by the way), then obviously society is going to
want to do something about it, and a nosy psychiatrist on a
grotty ward is a marginally kinder and more appropriate parallel
system than the norm for dangerous stuff, which is PC Plod and
his grotty cell. And if I were in serious danger of killing
myself, then God knows I would want someone to put me
somewhere safe and watch me like a hawk so that I could live

to see another day when the clouds had passed.

Perhaps you feel strongly about this: you are of absolutely sound mind right now (although take nothing for granted and be nice to the afflicted, because madness awaits us all). Perhaps, looking at the facts, you know that you would not want to be on a ward or on drugs in any circumstances. You would rather take your chances in that prison cell or maybe restrained instead of sedated like in America, or maybe you want to see how things go in your afterlife. And you know you definitely don't want ECT.

So make a living will. It is probably my only good idea ever.

I mean, mental illness of one kind or another has a lifetime incidence of well over 10 per cent: it is a hell of a lot more likely than your video recorder breaking down within three years. I can promise you it is a much better use of your time and money than that pricy extended warranty. This is, after all, your life we are talking about. You could maybe even mention how you feel about organ donation and being in a coma while you're at it, and save your family a whole lot of fretting.

After all, sometimes it feels as if all I ever do at parties is hold seminars defending the work of evil old psychiatry. People seem to cleave into either feckless buffoons who believe any infringement of liberties by a shrink is an act of patriarchal self-aggrandizement or those, usually with a palpable fear of their own madness, who want to know why on earth 'these people' are left to roam the streets lowering property prices.

'Shouldn't you be looking after them?' they ask, as I think of three good reasons to pour my drink over their heads.

Patients are nice people, like everyone else, and so are psychiatrists. We are doing our best, and we are probably doing the right thing, but Christ it feels grim sometimes.

If you feel so strongly about it either way, make a decision, make a living will, and try to get someone to take it seriously. And then maybe I can sleep easier at night, without that pleading, tearful face staring back at me.

Sophie's Nipples

Clearly the greatest joy of being a doctor is when your friends start asking you for help with their vile medical problems. Last week, for example, Sophie – the woman I have loved (unrequitedly) for more than a year – asked me about a lump in her breast.

Oh joy, I thought, as she described in detail the soft, fluctuant mass just lateral to her left nipple.

Of course, this only gets worse now that I'm a psychiatrist. My patchy knowledge of physical medicine has already receded, but worse than that, my friends are starting to ask questions about their mental health. Or even more hideously, the suicidal gestures of their partners.

You can see, I would hope, that there are at least eight million reasons why I would want to avoid these questions. The main one is that in most cases there are going to be a whole bunch of intrusive questions that I will need to ask.

I do not, at a party, want to ask about someone's bowel movements, nor do I want to start excluding a sexually transmitted disease as the cause of their symptoms in front of their faithful Christian girlfriend. The wisdom of this justification has, I like to imagine, been distilled into my stock response, which I can only recommend all doctors take up.

The conversation goes like this: 'Mike, do you know anything about that thing where you get a really sharp shooting pain across the bottom of your foot when you take your first steps in the morning?'

'Hmm,' I say, scratching the side of my head. 'Do you need a poo?'

It is the best response. It is, for a start, the only strategy that never fails to raise a smile among my puerile and hypochondriacal sisters, and can be deployed for any medical problem.

For example, last week on the bus: 'Mike, can I talk to you about Sam? He's drinking heavily. He becomes abusive and threatens to kill himself before vomiting everywhere.'

'Hmm,' I reply, scratching my head. 'Does he need a poo?'

Problem solved.

So, to return to Sophie's breasts: there is no way I'm going to sacrifice what little respect and affection she might have for me in the name of some cheap poo gag. No, I'm going to give this my best shot. I rack my brains for unsexual pathological data on breasts and try to be businesslike.

'Do you have a first-degree relative with breast cancer?'

'My mum almost died of breast cancer last year.'

Bollocks. This was something I had made big mileage out of, to my enormous shame. It wasn't just mileage, obviously. I mean, I'm not that low, and I love this girl as a friend, too. But I had a massive crush and it was a truly awful scene, and I was in the thick of it: the medical details seemed irrelevant. I never thought forgetting the physical pathology behind it would have such repercussions.

I flounder, trying to swerve us back to the neutrality of fact.

'Right,' I say, confidently. 'Your risk of getting it yourself is 13 per cent.'

'So what are they going to do at the appointment?'

'I guess they'll do an FNA.' God knows if that's true.

'What's an FNA?'

'They get a needle and stick it into your breast under ultra-sound guidance. Then they suck a bit of the fluid off the lump to see if it's cancer or not.'

'Great,' she says. 'Thanks.'

'I'm sure it'll be fine,' I say.

I'm probably wrong – about everything. I'm not a doctor. I'm just pretending. It's like those stories in the *Sun* about impostors with no medical degree. I'm just a sad, alcoholic fantasist who tells poo jokes.

Sophie starts to finish her drink.

'Look! Over there!' I blurt. 'Didn't he used to go out with Kylie?'

Epilogue

Writing Myself Out of a Job or How I Stopped Being an Arse

I guess I should explain why I stopped. If this was *EastEnders*, about now I'd have an affair and get run over by a car. The trite answer is that I started to love my job, and there is nothing more tedious than reading about a requited love affair. I was starting to be an all right psychiatrist, in a nice job: you can't write about that in 800-word anecdotes. And I didn't want to carry on just talking about the horrible stuff.

Although if you tied me down and held the ECT machine up to my genitals I could tell you what actually happened to me: I started child psychiatry and it turned my head upside down. Suddenly the blamelessness of psychiatric pathology is writ large in front of your eyes. And it's impossible to resent a child; unless, I guess, it's your own and you have to live with it.

You see a patient walk in to the room, in child psychiatry, with its parents, and suddenly you can see the punter – and I will use that word for paying customers until the day I die – as part of a system, its symptoms just a symptom of a family. Not that they're cursed by evil parents. It just all starts to seem a lot more complicated than just one person and a few chemicals.

And maybe it was that I finally had a nice boss.

But there's more than that. When you send a depressed child home, it goes home with two people who love it and want the best for it. When did I ever see that in adult psychiatry?

Looking back, I can't get over how persecuted I felt when I was a junior doctor. I think it's because, when you're a junior doctor, you really are persecuted. You have the frontline contact with the relatives; nurses are (and they really are) often absolutely horrible to you, for no good reason. You're working insane hours and no one is even vaguely sympathetic.

I suppose, for my own sanity, I ought to say something about the few people who wrote in to say that they were horrified by what I wrote. Remember that psychiatrists are all supposed to be weirdos, so if I was human that can't be such a bad thing. Although I hope it wasn't too awful. Or at least, if it was, I hope that you might understand why. Lots of people wrote very nice letters too, but sometimes I'd panic that people didn't need to know what nastiness can pass through the head of a junior doctor. From talking to other doctors, I reassured myself that it was fairly representative, not of what it's like to be a doctor but of what it's like to be a new doctor, often working in situations where you felt very unsupported. I was once at a party where a medical student said she thought Foxton was 'a bit harsh'. How cruelly we laughed.

But, most importantly, and this really is important to me, I hope that I didn't, as a couple of people suggested, imply that all psychiatric patients were violent when I wrote honestly about feeling a bit scared – unnecessarily as it turned out – by one patient very early on. I've got on very well with most of my patients; they're the main reason I'm in the trade. And it's Ok to have feelings: in fact that was the title of a handout that someone sent me from their medical school lectures that used my columns as case material. That seems to have happened a lot and, in my own cheesy way, I was moved to hear that the column on suicide was used in one place as the parting note before they sent their baby doctors out alone into the hellish world of medicine. Do come back if you need a chat is a very important thing to say to people who are that alone, and I wish someone had said it more forcefully to the doctor I knew who killed himself.

Of course, one big problem for your head, when you're a junior doctor, is that you move every six months, just when you're putting down roots. Of course, this can sometimes be a very good thing. I cannot even begin to describe the messiness of my six months as a surgical house officer: it was like a Channel 5 soap opera about doctors and nurses sleeping with each other. I remember sitting in my room, at one in the morning, having to turn up the stereo to prevent an anaesthetist from the same hospital hearing the sound of his wife fucking my dear friend Dr Winnicott very loudly in the on-call room next door. I remember the entire on-call ward round being led by the consultant over to Bedside Manor to find me, on the day of my one and only hangover-related day-off, in bed with the loveliest medical SHO in the hospital. For six months we drank until we vomited and then gave each other drips, anti-emetics, painkillers and ulcer drugs to get through the next day without collapsing. And I never saw any of these people more than twice in the next two years.

These were the things that kept me sane, and made me happy. Now the things that make me happy are my girlfriend who will soon be my wife, and the babies I plan to have, and the chance that I might one day get better at being a shrink. I don't want to make my work into funny stories, and I don't need to any more, because you know it all now. I'm a psychiatrist. Not a writer. And I hope I'll be an all right one.

Appendix or, Sliced Liver, Anyone?

Anatomy, I have to admit, bored me senseless at medical school. So I was secretly quite pleased, at the first public autopsy in 170 years, to stick firmly with tradition and show up five minutes late, after smoking a cigarette outside the back of the lecture theatre.

I found it hard to imagine what could possibly be exciting about this event, having sat through a year of unremittingly tedious dissection classes. But one thing kept my interest. We were apparently to witness the autopsy of a thirty-three-year-old German woman with epilepsy: and her parents, who would be in the audience, hoped to discover whether their daughter had committed suicide and whether she was pregnant.

Even from a culture with a proven track record in embarrassing openness and excessive public nudity, this seemed a little too close to *Jerry Springer* for comfort. It's hard to think of anything less British than the denouement on your daughter's suicide coming in front of an audience of 300 strangers, but here we all were; and there at the front, under a white sheet, was a real live dead person.

Professor Gunther von Hagens seems rather pleased with his infamy. He invented plastination, a technique for preserving dead body parts, and has now found fame peddling Body Worlds, an art exhibition of preserved corpses in exotic poses. This has alarmed and excited in equal measure, but now – apparently in response to a legal threat of closure – he has announced his intention to perform this public spectacle. This, we are told, is part of his mission to democratize access to the mysteries of the body, previously the domain of the 'profesional medical élite'. Gunther, apparently, is a radical. I, at the tender age of twenty-six, am a member of the élite.

Sadly, we are told, there has been a change of plan. He will be dissecting a man in his seventies who has apparently died of heart failure. He was an alcoholic, apparently, on two bottles of whisky a day, and he failed to work much beyond the age of fifty. The audience – consisting of art students, London trendies, everyday folk in anoraks and at least a million journalists – when presented with this unnecessary biographical information, simultaneously gasp with a disapproving and noisy intake of breath.

A German pathologist speaks: 'You, the eagerly awaiting public, will now witness the dissection of a human body!' I can tell you, we didn't get that level of showmanship at medical school. 'What is crucial,' he announces in reverent tones, 'is maintaining respect for the human body.'

Two men behind me start to giggle as the sheet is pulled away, and suddenly I am very glad we are not dissecting a young woman. Are they laughing at his willy?

Gunther cuts down into the man's chest and on towards the abdomen, tearing away the skin from the chest wall.

Nobody winces. Nobody vomits. Nobody leaves.

He gestures expansively to the audience and announces that he will take questions from his 'students', 'as I move down the abdomen to –' (the giggling men behind me finish the sentence '– his nuts!')

'I don't understand why only scientists can have access to the inside of the human body,' explains Gunther as he pulls apart the tissue to leave sheets of skin lying either side of the man's open chest.

I stop to think. The process of dismemberment is a deeply weird and dysphoric experience, and it's a dangerous border to cross. We have, quite rightly, an intuitive respect for human bodies, and the value of keeping sharp knives away from them.

I remember the first time I had to cross that boundary, as a medical student in an operating theatre. It was a man with stomach cancer, whom I had been talking to on the ward the morning before his operation. When the surgeon brought down the knife to make the first cut on his belly, it was everything I could do to stop myself reaching out and grabbing his hand to stop him. Something deep inside me was saying: What the hell does that bloke think he's doing with that knife?

Doctors have to cross that boundary. We have to separate the thinking, smiling, family man from the clinical material. If I hadn't done that, I couldn't possibly cut a hole and force a huge chest-drain tube a centimetre across into a writhing patient on a respiratory ward at 3 a.m. without going mad.

But maybe you don't all need to start thinking like that. Later, when he cuts the brain with a big flat surgical knife, Gunter says that it can easily be substituted, if you are short of money, with a salmon knife, for just £11, from any store. This is surely the wrong message. I'd have preferred 'Don't try this at home, kids.'

A doctor in the audience has a question: 'What were the clinical observations at the time of death?'

The team of pathologists fudge. 'Probably he would have been short of breath,' says one.

The doctor repeats his question.

'He would have had difficulty climbing the stairs,' says another.

'No,' says the doctor. 'What were the heart sounds? What did the doctors hear with a stethoscope in the chest? What was the white cell count?'

Nobody knows.

We could all, apparently, be told that he was a person who lost his job to alcohol, but not the most basic clinical information. Some post-mortem. Some educational experience. I can't even begin to imagine the hammering I'd have got, as a junior doctor, not knowing the answers to questions like these. But the showmen professors do not seem embarrassed.

Gunther begins to peel back the scalp like a big wet flappy wig – there's a graphic tearing sound as he pulls it away – and takes a bandsaw to the skull; legs akimbo and his knees bent. It's a fantastic noise, combining the nastiness of fingernails on a blackboard with the knowledge that it's the sound of a renegade German anatomist sawing someone's skull open. Everybody loves it, and literally half the audience is giggling.

Three young women in my stall walk out. Something squirts. It is at least nine months since I had to remember to keep my mouth shut in a situation like this. An assistant takes over as Gunther moves back to remove the bodily organs that his minions have teased loose. He lifts out the lungs and tells us the man was a smoker, to more disapproval. When he lifts the abdominal contents they are very heavy, and when he finally manages to heave them out he gets a round of applause. And that applause (not his first or his last) is perhaps the strangest thing.

I cannot help wondering whether Gunther feels outdone by his corpses. Is that what this autopsy is all about? He has made a world famous 'art' exhibition, but the beauty is all in the human body. Where was the place for Gunther in all this, before the big show?

That's certainly how it looks in the promotional photograph that's been in all the newspapers: two partially dismembered corpses in the foreground, on either side of Gunther, stare ahead disinterestedly, while he puts his arms matily round their shoulders and grins, hoping we can all see what great mates they are. The corpses know they're the show: they don't care about Gunther. But Gunther wants a piece of the action.

Mercifully it's half-time. I'm starving, and suddenly I remember how hungry dissection class always used to make us. Three times a week there was the familiar rush for the chicken sandwiches in the biochemistry department canteen. Although because our impoverished medical school could never afford rubber gloves for all of us, we always had to pick our nails clean first.

I chat to some of the punters. My first question, of course, is why did you come?

'I've got no spleen.'

'Really?' I ask.

'Really.' She lifts her jumper to reveal an enormous scar on her abdomen. I make my excuses and ask someone else.

'I'm a masseur, so I've got to know about anatomy.'

'Is this any help?' I ask.

'No,' she says, beaming, 'but you'll never see that again, will you?'

I make it my mission to find someone earnest. I eavesdrop on a couple talking about how it demystified death and helped them to understand anatomy. Had either of them ever looked at an anatomy textbook?

'No, but I've read lots of fiction.' I wait. 'You know, horror novels.'

They ask why I'm here. I tell them I'm a doctor. They ask if I've seen it all before. 'It used to bore me senseless,' I say, 'and it always started at eight in the morning.'

They look at me like I'm the freak.

And then I find her. A girl who is such a fan she has signed up to donate her body.

'I saw Gunther at the airport and ran over to tell him how much I respected his work,' she says. 'There are only three other girls my age who are donors.'

'You've met them?'

'Oh sure, but I missed the free trip to China. I was well miffed.'

I've read about Gunther's place in China. Plastination City: fifty Chinese anatomists all working in one room for £180 a month. It sounds a bit like a sweatshop. He has previously said that the part of the world that gave us exquisite calligraphy is full of top dissectors. I remember that I'm pretending to be a journalist today.

'Do you mind if I put you in an article?' I ask.

'Oh sure. I'm already in the *Mail* and the *Standard*.'

I keep my mouth shut. I think I might find it rather belittling to die and be reincarnated as a walk-on part in The Gunther Show.

We go back in for part two, in which Gunther and the other pathologists talk us through various organs laid out on metal dishes. Someone starts to talk about atherosclerosis in the aorta – now I'm really struggling to stay awake. He lists the risk factors for cardiovascular disease. I begin to nod off; even the audience is getting restless, and I am struck by a Proustian rush: I am thrown into the mists of time, sitting in the dark at the back of the anatomy lecture theatre at medical school, trying to chat up Sarah Hawking all over again.

Someone passes round a dish of sliced liver. Now I'm ravenous.

It's almost over. Gunther, the showman, gets called away to do a crucial television interview. The other pathologists begin to field dry 'educational' questions from the audience. And this is the most telling moment of the evening: because at least a quarter of the audience drifts away.

The only British pathologist begs them to stay. People have debated the morality of this evening's event and, out of respect for the dead, to demonstrate the educational value of the event, he pleads, we should stay to the end. People continue to leave. The star has gone. The fireworks are spent. Now it's just a pathology lecture. And you really don't need me to tell you how boring they are.